Secrets of the

drugs

industry

Bryan Hubbard

D0293827

A What Doctors Don't Tell You publication

500 838889

First published in Great Britain in 2002 by WDDTY Ltd., 2 Salisbury Road, London SW19 4EZ

ISBN 0-9534734-6-5
Cover illustration: Louise Chavannes

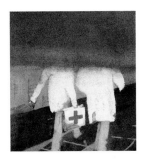

CONTENTS

CONTENTS (continued)

(Accolate; Adalat; Adifax; Aricept; Asacol; aspirin; Baycol;
Becloforte; Betaferon; Bricanyl; Brufen; Burinex; Cardura;
Ciproxin; Claritin; Clomid; Condrotec; Cordarone; Cozaar;
Desmospray; Dexedrine; Didronel; Diflucan; Dutonin; Efexor;
Eltroxin; Emblon; Epilim; Evista; Feldene; Fosamax; Genticin;
Imigran; Imuran; Lamictal; Lamisil; Larim; L-Dopa; Lipostat;
Livial; Losec; Lotronex; Lustral; Manerix; Marevan; Megace;
Minocin; Neotigason; Nicotinell; Nivaquine; Ortho-Gynest;
Phenergan; Plaquenil; Plavix; Pondimin; Posicor; Premarin;
Prepulsid; Proscar; Prozac; Pulmicort; PumpHep; Questran;
Rapamune; Relenza; Relpax; Retin-A; Rezulin; Rifater; Ritalin;
Roaccutane; Roferon-A; Roxiam; Sandimmune; Septrin;
Seretide; Serevent; Seroxat; Sporanox; Tegretol; Ticlid;
Triludan; Viagra; Vioxx; Xenical; Zantac; Zestril; Zimovane;
Zocor; Zorac; Zoton; Zovirax; Zydol)

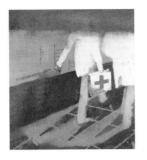

INTRODUCTION

*I*n recent times, AIDS and murder have rarely been off the front pages; not surprisingly, perhaps, as they are two of the major ills of our society.

Pop stars Elton John and Michael Jackson have been joining forces with film celebrity Elizabeth Taylor to raise the public awareness of AIDS, and to loosen the public purse strings so that more funding can be found for research into a cure. Similarly, politicians and police chiefs have been wrestling over a series of measures—including after-hours clubs at schools, liberalisation of the softer drugs, and on-the-spot fines—to try and reduce violent crime that can so easily lead to murder.

Their concerns are well placed. In one year in America alone, around 13,500 people are murdered, and 13,000 die from AIDS. Combined, that would be like the population of a reasonable-sized town in the UK just disappearing every year.

But there is something even more astonishing that leaps off the page when you scan the causes of death of any country. It's like a silent killer that never attracts the headlines, never interests the politicians or the pop stars—it's death from prescription drugs. For the same period in the US, 113,000 people died either as a reaction to a drug or because of an error in medication. Interestingly, this latter group amounts to just 7,000 of the total, so that means the vast majority suffered what is euphemistically called "an adverse reaction" to the medication that had been prescribed by a doctor.

It's been likened to a jumbo jet crashing every day of the year, killing over 300 passengers each time. As a matter of interest, the situation concerning all of medicine is even worse. At least 225,000 die in the US as a direct result of conventional medicine going wrong, making it the third major killer in the West after heart disease and cancer.

A similar picture can be painted in the UK. The Medicines Control Agency (MCA), which monitors the safety of drugs after they reach the market, reported that, in the year 2000, 33,109 adverse reactions to drugs were reported, of which 14,500 were serious, and 600 were fatal.

Perhaps those figures represent more of the image of a world we believe we live in, one where we can trust those in positions of authority to ensure our safety and wellbeing. Unfortunately, the figures cannot be relied on. The UK in particular, and Europe in general, suffer from a massive underreporting of drug side effects and adverse reactions. It's impossible to measure what is not known, but it's been reckoned that just 1 per cent of adverse reactions are reported to the American drug regulator, the Food and Drug Administration (FDA), and a similar estimate could be applied here. One French study found that just 1 out of every 20,000 reactions to prescription drugs is ever reported. Dr Bill Inman, who created the UK's Yellow Card system of reporting drug reactions in 1963, does not believe the problem is quite that bad, but accepts that only around 10 per cent of all reactions is ever reported. Whichever estimate you take, the true picture is clearly far more shocking than any of us imagine, and indeed should be the stuff of national, and international, scandal.

Quite why this appalling state of affairs is allowed to continue without comment or control is the subject of this report, but it's worth saying here that we live in a culture that recognises the hard work of doctors and hospital staffs, and the fact that everyone is doing their best in difficult circumstances. And, of course, nobody wanted these people to die; quite the reverse, in fact.

Each death is also lonely and quiet; there's no blazing

wreckage, no buildings collapsing. Just people, mainly elderly, dying in a bed, or suffering some reaction that cripples their lives, but getting nobody to admit blame.

If a similar situation were allowed to continue in the airline industry, nobody would fly again until the problem was recognised and rectified.

Unfortunately, patients don't enjoy the same choice. They have to take the drugs that they've been prescribed, and are quietly hopeful that all the controls are in place and that the drug they are about to take is safe, or reasonably so.

If, taking a very conservative estimate, drugs are killing 113,000 Americans every year, this is not a reasonable assumption to take.

This report endeavours to explain why this is happening, not so that you should come off the course of treatment you may already be on, but so you can ask more intelligent questions and thus reduce the risk of your joining the ballooning ranks of victims that nobody will acknowledge.

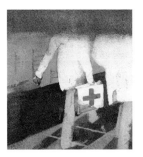

CHAPTER ONE *NOT MANY DEAD...*

I t was the end of another busy week at the offices of What Doctors Don't Tell You, and everyone was keen to get their coats on and head for home for the weekend. Just then the phone rang, and each person looked to the next as if to say: "Why don't you answer it?" In the end, one staff member picked up the receiver to hear a message he would never forget.

The voice at the other end was a woman's. She explained that, on that very day, she had retired from a fairly senior position at a drug company. She refused to reveal which one. She said she was so relieved to leave her job. "I just got tired of sweeping things under the carpet. The number of deaths caused by our drugs is appalling. It has been like working for a morgue." At that she hung up, perhaps relieved that her confession had somehow made her heart a little lighter, and her retirement a little happier.

For us, it was a frustrating call. The tone of her voice suggested she had been genuine; anyone who wanted to mislead us would have given us much more information than the tantalising nuggets she did impart. Perhaps she didn't know any more than that, although the way she had spoken suggested this was unlikely.

We hadn't been producing What Doctors Don't Tell You that long when she made her call, but hers was not the first pointer that all was not quite right in the state of the pharmaceutical industry.

All those years later, we know she was speaking the truth. What we still don't know is the actual size of the problem, although it must be far worse than the official figures that paint a scary enough picture.

What we do know is that at least 106,000 Americans die every year as a result of some adverse reaction (ADR) to a prescription drug, and a further 7,000 die from an error relating to a drug, such as a wrong dosage or the wrong concoction. We know this because the Institute of Medicine (IOM) carried out a survey among patients who died while in an American hospital. This startling piece of research was published in the prestigious Journal of the American Medical Association (JAMA, 2000; 284: 2184–5).

These figures are just the tip of the iceberg. Many, many people die from a reaction to a drug, but a link is never established; many, many people die in their homes rather than in hospital, or report their symptoms as an outpatient or to their family doctor. Finally, the vast majority of drug-related deaths are never reported at all. In concluding its research paper, the IOM accepted that its findings were a gross undercalculation for those very reasons.

It's worth stressing that we are talking solely about deaths; the numbers of people who are seriously harmed, possibly for life, by a drug are not even touched upon in the study.

In all, 225,000 people in the USA die every year as a result of medicine, and drugs are the cause of half of all these deaths, says the IOM.

This was not an isolated finding. Another study from the University of South Alabama College of Medicine, published three years earlier, reckoned that 180,000 people die in American hospitals every year, but again admitted that the figure could well be a serious underestimate. Unlike the IOM's, this study also calculates that around one million people are injured while in an American hospital (Am Fam Physician, 1997; 56: 1781–8).

A similar gloomy picture is painted in the UK, although scaled down because of the smaller population. Here, medical errors, which include drug reactions, kill 40,000 people every year, according to a study by the University College London. Again, the study is based on deaths in hospitals and so excludes the many more deaths that happen at home.

All the research teams emphasise the problems of under-reporting because it is an enormous issue that masks the real picture. The reasons tend to be human rather than sinister. Sometimes the link between a death and a drug is not reported because no test up to that time had realised that the reaction could be fatal. If it's not documented already, it's not going to be noted. Sometimes the doctor forgets to report it, or just puts it to one side along with the pile of paperwork he already has to do sometime. And, in a very few cases, the real cause is deliberately hidden.

To take one example, the Food and Drug Administration, the USA's drug regulator, receives around 82 cases a year of adverse reactions among patients taking digoxin, the heart drug. However, a quick scan of the papers of Medicare, the health insurance scheme in America, discovered there were 202,211 cases over seven years—an average of 28,887 a year—where the patient received hospital care after reacting to the drug (JAMA, 1998; 279: 1571–3).

French researchers reached similar findings. They reckon that doctors report only one in 24,433 adverse reactions. They based their shocking conclusion on a study of 100 doctors practising in the Bordeaux area of France, and compared their adverse drug reporting level to reports received at the Bordeaux drug monitoring centre from doctors not participating in the study (Br J Clin Pharmacol, 1997; 43: 177–81).

Dr Bill Inman, who started the Yellow Card system in the UK in 1963, has made the most conservative view of the level of underreporting. The system is simple enough; if a GP suspects a drug has caused an adverse reaction, he writes it down on the Yellow Card and sends it back to the Medicines Control Agency, the UK group that monitors the safety of drugs once they are licensed. Dr Inman reckons just 10 per cent of all reactions are ever reported, again because a link is either never suspected, or because the GP is already awash with an enormous backlog of forms to complete.

So, whether it's 1 in 24,433 cases or 1 in 352 (extrapolated from the digoxin example), or if it's Dr Inman's 1 in 10 best guess, the situation is clearly far worse than the official figures suggest.

The Medicines Control Agency says that 33,109 adverse reactions to drugs were reported to its officials in 2000, which was 55 per cent up on 1999. Of these, 44 per cent were serious reactions, and 2 per cent were fatal. According to those figures, 600 people in Britain died as a result of a drug reaction in 2000.

But if we apply even the most conservative estimate of underreporting, this would mean that around 6,000 people died in the UK from an adverse drug reaction in the year; apply the Medicare digoxin analysis and the true death tally balloons to a figure in excess of 200,000. By comparison, fewer than 500 people die in the UK every year from AIDS, so even if the MCA statistics are accepted at face value, drugs are a bigger killer in the UK than AIDS.

Thus far, we've been looking only at fatalities, which is the least common reaction of them all, of course. Let's now turn to what is described as a 'serious' adverse reaction. This would usually mean the immediate stopping of the drug therapy, provided the doctor realises that the drug is the problem. As we've already seen, that can be a big 'if'. A serious reaction, as defined by medicine, usually results in permanent disability or, at the very least, a stay in hospital.

One study found that 2,216,000 Americans suffer a serious reaction—that is, they are permanently disabled or spend time in hospital—from a prescribed drug every year (JAMA, 1998; 279: 1200–5). This doesn't include the many others who suffer a bad reaction that doesn't leave them permanently disabled, or who are treated as outpatients.

This also doesn't allow for the problem of underreporting. Most of the analysis of underreporting we've looked at so far relates to GPs. So what about underreporting at hospitals? The same problem seems to apply. Researchers reckon that hospital consultants report only 1 in 20 adverse reactions, sometimes because they fear a lawsuit (JAMA, 1998; 279: 1216–7).

One study concluded that there are 88 things that can go wrong when a doctor fills out a prescription in hospital, and all the mistakes could be fatal. A research team from the University of London asked the pharmacists at a 550-bed teaching hospital to inform them whenever there was a potentially serious prescribing error. In all, they identified 88 over a two-month period—with 50 of them committed by one junior doctor.

When questioned later, the doctors blamed the errors on tiredness, being distracted or sheer ignorance of the drug and dosage they were prescribing. One doctor was unaware that the drug he prescribed was linked to kidney failure. Worse, he admitted that he did not know how to diagnose kidney failure if it happened or what to do about the drug when kidney failure was diagnosed, presumably by another doctor (Lancet, 2002; 359: 1373–8).

In the UK, the MCA is aware of 33,109 ADRs reported in 2000, of which 44 per cent were "serious". That means, even according to the official figures, that drugs permanently disabled 14,500 people that year. If we then use the most conservative model of underreporting, the true figure reaches close to 150,000. However, research at University College London, led by Charles Vincent, suggests the real figure is closer to 280,000 people suffering a serious reaction every year in the UK. The reaction is usually severe enough to warrant up to six days' hospital treatment, which translates to 1,680,000 hospital bed-days a year, causing an enormous strain on an already overstretched National Health Service.

The problem is partly to do with multiple prescriptions to elderly patients. Another major factor is the constant release of new drugs into the marketplace, a drive more to do with a drug company's share price than the benefit of mankind, as we shall see.

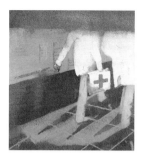

CHAPTER TWO *NEW DRUGS FOR OLD*

Pharmaceuticals make up the most profitable industry sector in the world. In the year 2000, the top 20 drug companies had a combined sale of £135 billion, and they enjoyed an average growth rate of 11 per cent. Sales topped £155 billion in 2001, double the revenues achieved in 1997.

The overall profitability of pharmaceuticals was further emphasised in the Fortune 500 list. While the average Fortune 500 company saw profits during 2001 nosedive by 53 per cent, the drug companies on the list saw theirs leap another 33 per cent.

Collectively, the top 10 drug companies in the list topped all three of the magazine's measures of profitability. They enjoyed the greatest return on revenues, reporting a profit of 18.5 cents for every $1 of sales, which was eight times higher than the combined return of every other sector on the list. Commercial banking achieved a return of just 13.5 cents per $1 made.

During the year, the pharmaceutical giants' advertising expenditure outstripped major retail manufacturers such as Nike, while spending far less than expected on research.

Britain's largest drug company—and the second largest in the world after Pfizer—is GlaxoSmithKline (GSK) which, in 2001, achieved sales of £20.5 billion, and a pretax profit of £6.2 billion, an astonishing margin of 31 per cent. The GSK figures confirm the Fortune findings that the pharmaceutical industry is by far the most profitable in the world, outstripping the automobile, petrochemical, property, banking and technology sectors with ease (N Engl J Med, 2000; 342: 1902–4).

The major lifeblood for any industry, and this is especially true for drug companies, is new product. Shareholders and city analysts alike thirst for news of new breakthroughs, cures for disease X, and so on. It's what drives the share price, and keeps investor interest strong.

The problem is that it can cost a pharmaceutical company anything up to £350 million to successfully bring a new drug to market. It's also very hit-and-miss, with plenty of false trails before the research chemists feel they are finally on to something.

It's been estimated that it can take from 10 to 15 years from that first "eureka" moment until the drug is finally licensed for use, and that just three out of 10 drug companies ever recoup all

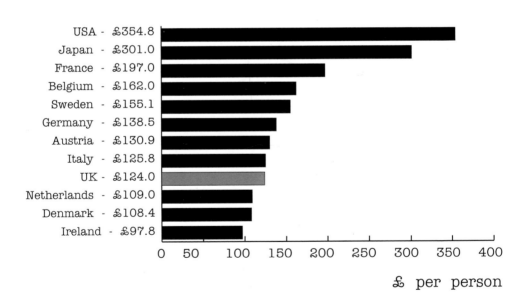

Annual medicine usage per person

	£ per person
USA - £354.8	
Japan - £301.0	
France - £197.0	
Belgium - £162.0	
Sweden - £155.1	
Germany - £138.5	
Austria - £130.9	
Italy - £125.8	
UK - £124.0	
Netherlands - £109.0	
Denmark - £108.4	
Ireland - £97.8	

£ per person

Notes: £ per person includes prescription and hospital medicines
Source: IMS World Review 2001 United Nations, World
population Prospects Office for National Statistics
ABPI

Leading pharmaceutical corporations, 2000

	Country	Sales £m	Growth[a] %	World market share[b] %
Pfizer	USA	15,266	13	7.3
GlaxoSmithKline	UK	14,533	13	6.9
Merck & Co	USA	10,875	18	5.2
AstraZeneca	UK	9,423	11	4.5
Bristol-Myers Squibb	USA	8,758	12	4.2
Novartis	SWI	8,187	7	3.9
Johnson & Johnson	USA	8,152	13	3.9
Aventis	FRA	7,457	5	3.6
Pharmacia	USA	6,758	15	3.2
American Home Products	USA	6,310	11	3.0
Leading 10		**95,721**	**12**	**45.7**
Eli Lilly	USA	6,149	11	2.9
Roche	SWI	6,103	4	2.9
Abbott	USA	5,153	5	2.5
Schering-Plough	USA	5,104	6	2.4
Bayer	GER	4,059	8	1.9
Takeda	JAP	3,691	29	1.8
Boehringer Ingelheim	GER	2,906	11	1.4
Sanofi-Synthélabo	FRA	2,403	9	1.1
Amgen	USA	2,028	9	1.0
Schering AG	GER	1,941	5	0.9
Leading 20		**135,258**	**11**	**64.6**

Notes:
By worldwide sales value
[a] Calculated in local currencies; [b] IMS audited markets = 87% of all markets and includes top 60 by value
Source: IMS ABPI

the development costs of bringing a new drug to market. Despite the risks, most drug companies are pursuing the pharmacy's Holy Grail—the next magic bullet.

The importance of new product lines for the pharmaceutical industry cannot be overstressed; in the USA in 2000, 33.7 per cent of all drug prescriptions were for new products, closely followed by the Canadian market, where new drugs accounted for 29.8 per cent of all sales. In the UK, new drugs represented 15.7 per cent of the total market.

This market share is mirrored in revenues. Turning again to GlaxoSmithKline as an example, new products represented 22 per cent of total pharmaceutical sales in 2001. In all, the conglomerate introduced 10 new products into development during the year.

The pharmaceutical companies argue that new product research is essential to combat disease, a view that, to an extent, is true. But the argument only has validity if it can be shown that existing drugs on the market cannot perform equally as well; unfortunately, this is a question that is rarely asked.

It's also worth noting that, while drug companies like to see themselves as altruistic champions of mankind, most spend twice as much on marketing and advertising as they do on research. This is another symptom of the licensing process. A patent, usually running for 20 years, is taken out once the research team has made an initial breakthrough. However, once the licensing process has been completed, the patent may have only another five or six years left to run before other drug companies can produce 'me-too' copies. This means the drug company has only a short window of time to recoup its £350 million initial investment, and so embarks on a very aggressive marketing campaign from the outset.

Drug companies are also not as innovative as they'd have us believe. The high costs of research tend to prevent highly experimental work. Most new drugs are modifications of existing ones. Dr John Griffin, then a senior official in the medicines division at the Department of Health, discovered in a study he conducted in 1981 that the 204 new chemical entities (NCEs) marketed over the previous decade had largely been introduced into areas

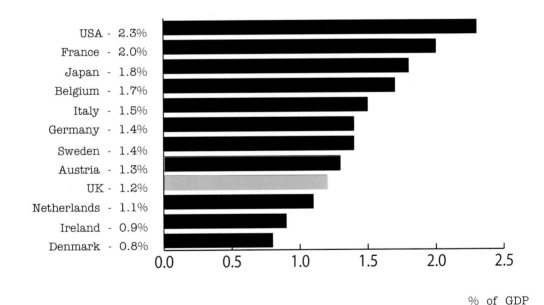

Spend on medicine as a percentage of GDP in various countries, 2000

% of GDP

Notes: Includes prescription and hospital medicines
Source: IMS World Review 2001 ABPI

"already heavily oversubscribed", he said. "Innovation is directed towards commercial returns rather than therapeutic need."

Later research suggests that nothing has changed. A study in America discovered that, of all the drugs approved during the 1990s, only 15 per cent contained new active ingredients, and could be viewed as a significant improvement over existing drugs on the market.

The study, produced by the National Institute for Health Care Management (NIHCM) Foundation, reviewed the 1,035 prescription drugs approved by the Food and Drug Administration (FDA), the American drug regulator, between 1989 and 2000. Only one-third, or 361 drugs, were new molecular entities, which treat diseases in novel ways, the investigators found. Less than half of these drugs were given priority status by the FDA, a special category for drugs that the agency believes could provide significant clinical improvement over existing medications.

Among the innovative drugs were Pfizer's Lipitor (atorvastatin) for high cholesterol, and Viagra (sildenafil) for erectile dysfunction; Merck & Co's Fosamax (alendronate sodium) for osteoporosis, and GlaxoSmithKline's Avandia (rosiglitazone) for type II diabetes.

Of the rest, 674 drugs approved during the 10-year period contained active ingredients that were already available in drugs that had been previously approved. In other words, they were 'me-too' drugs. The only difference in most cases was either a different dosage, or a new added ingredient. A drug, previously only available in oral form, might instead be available as a transdermal patch, for instance.

So why go to the expense and bother of creating a 'new' drug that adds nothing to the wellbeing of mankind? Apart from the effect that a new drug can have on the share price, drug companies can also charge more for the new drug. The NIHCM study found that all new drugs were priced much higher than the old ones they were endevouring to replace. In America in 2000, the average price per prescription for the most innovative class of drugs was $91.20 versus an average price of $37.20 for older dugs that were approved before 1995.

Even the 'me-too' drugs also commanded a higher price. On average, the more recently approved drug, which was virtually the same as an existing drug, cost around 75 per cent more than older drugs that provided an almost identical function.

This trend is continuing. The total spend on prescription drugs in the USA in 2000, the last year under review by the NIHCM study, was $132 billion. This rose in 2001 to $175 billion, and it is set to reach $200 billion in 2002.

The drug companies may argue that the extra revenues are needed to support research into new drugs—but if the so-called new offerings are identical to existing ones, it would seem that much of R&D in the pharmaceutical industry is done merely to boost share prices and revenues.

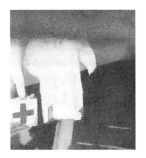

CHAPTER THREE *TESTING, TESTING...*

Marcia Angell, former editor-in-chief of the prestigious medical publication the New England Journal of Medicine once wrote: "To rely on the drug companies for unbiased evaluations of their products makes about as much sense as relying on beer companies to teach us about alcoholism" (N Engl J Med, 2000; 342: 1902–4).

That, unfortunately, is pretty much what we do rely on for assessing the safety of a new drug. And it must be remembered that there's immense pressure on a drug company to successfully bring a new drug to market—pressure from shareholders and city analysts, and the in-house pressures to recoup the vast investment involved. Success—not safety or efficacy—is therefore the single most important driving factor.

It took until the 1960s and the thalidomide scandal before it was recognised that greater drug controls were needed in the UK. This became even more pressing when it was discovered that the drug company concerned in the scandal had evidence of the possible risk of deformities before it released the drug.

In 1968, Britain introduced the Medicines Act to regulate the introduction of new drugs. The Medicines Commission was established a year later, and its task was to approve new drugs until it was replaced by the Medicines Control Agency in 1988.

The Committee on Safety of Medicines, which controls all drugs once on the market, was set up in 1970, followed in 1975 by the Committee on the Review of Medicines.

To prove its safety, quality and efficacy, a drug has to pass through several stages before a licence to market is granted. The first stage usually involves a very small group of healthy volunteers so scientists can understand how the compound metabolises, and so on. In phase two, a larger group, possibly up to 100 people suffering from the disease that the new medicine is designed to treat, are given the drug to see if it helps their condition. The third stage is the most exhaustive and expensive, and involves clinical trials. A test group has been as small as 18 people, but usually is about 1500 strong. This is a remarkably low number compared with the hundreds of thousands who will unwittingly test the drug once it has received a licence. For obvious reasons, it is also rare for a clinical trial to include children, pregnant women and the elderly, the very people who may suffer side effects once the drug is on the market. Taking part in a drugs trial is usually a good way for strapping young medical students to earn some extra money. They're also far less likely to suffer an adverse reaction than would a frail man of 80, who is probably also taking three or four other prescription drugs.

Some adverse reactions are immediate; often, though, they can take a while to appear, but this would never be discovered from the early trials.

Dosage is a key part of the safety picture. For example, women prescribed the birth-control pill in the 1960s were receiving between three and eight times the levels of oestrogen needed to prevent conception; those levels have now been seen to put a woman at a far higher risk of developing breast cancer (JAMA, 2000; 283: 485–91).

If the aim is to bring a drug to market, the researchers must establish the level of dose needed for the drug to work, and with as few serious adverse reactions as possible. However, few ask if the drug would still work at even lower doses.

The clinical trial sometimes involves a placebo (sugar pill) that is tested against it. There are no requirements laid down for the drug company to meet: it can determine how many people should be involved in the trial, whether to use a placebo, or whether the test should be a 'double-blind' (where the test subjects are split into groups receiving either the placebo or the drug and neither participants nor researchers are aware of which is being given).

With such lax guidelines, it's little wonder that Sir William Asscher, former chairman of the Committee on Safety of Medicines, in a private meeting, said: ". . . by the time a drug is licensed, we really know very little in the case of a new chemical entity about its possible risks." Despite this knowledge gap, the Medicines Control Agency prides itself on being the fastest regulator in Europe, granting a licence on average within 70 days, so making Britons the world's guinea pigs.

Some tests are aborted early if the responses seem particularly favourable, as happened with the anti-AIDS drug AZT, later discredited in the Concorde tests.

A number of drugs are also granted licences in the UK while being rejected or delayed a licence in the US. One example of this was the drug Centoxin, created by its US manufacturer Centocor to treat blood poisoning. The FDA had refused it a licence, but the UK granted one in May 1991. It was suddenly withdrawn in January 1993 when further studies from the US showed "excess mortality" among patients who did not have a certain type of blood poisoning. By the time this discovery was made, 2000 Britons had taken the drug, although no deaths had been reported at the time.

Sometimes, trials are not what they seem. One, which was testing an experimental cancer drug, resulted in the deaths of a number of patients. The drug company was paying the researchers involved for the number of patients they could 'recruit' to the trial. Presumably, the extent of the risk was never explained to the volunteers who took part in the fatal test.

In another trial, a healthy 18-year-old student died because of an experimental drug. Her family had not been told that the principal research scientist stood to profit if the drug had worked.

One early-stage trial, involving a group of university students, was for a drug laced with an industrial pollutant. Unfortunately, none of the students had been told of the deadly cocktail in the drug, nor were they told that the manufacturer was already being sued over the safety of the drug they were being asked to test.

In another study, a cancer research centre in America recruited volunteers to test a new drug. The doctors involved failed to tell the recruits that previous volunteers had died while testing the drug, and that they had a direct financial interest in the success of the drug (Lancet, 2002; 359: 1167).

To ease a drug through the licensing process, drug companies have sometimes designed the study to make the drug look more effective and less toxic. According to a 1994 study that appeared in the Archives of Internal Medicine, 54 per cent of trials into an arthritis drug found that the trial dose used was higher than that of a competing company's product, increasing the likelihood that the drug being tested would look more effective.

In another test, this time on a diabetes drug, the manufacturer hid data showing that the drug could cause liver failure. The drug was therefore granted a licence, but was withdrawn when it was suspected of causing the deaths of 391 patients.

Once a drug has been licensed, the drug company has only one legal requirement in Britain: to advertise the drug name, licence number and manufacturer details in an obscure official journal called the London Gazette. In the US, the FDA prints chapter and verse on its reasons for granting the licence; in the case of the antidepressant Prozac, for example, these reasons fill 48 pages, which are freely available to the general public. Under the Freedom of Information Act in the US, the FDA can disclose over 90 per cent of its records. Ironically, 85 per cent of requests for information come from the pharmaceutical industry itself, which opposes similar access in the UK. In the UK, the deliberations of the UK's Medicines Control Agency are kept secret, and no government minister or official can publish any information it finds out about a drug company or its research. Any breach of this law can result in two years' imprisonment. This extraordinary state of affairs, the most extreme protection enjoyed by any industry group, is enshrined in Section 118 of the 1968 Medicines Act, a section originally designed to protect commercial secrets, but which is used as a blanket ban on all information, including that which the public should have a right to know. It "protects" the public from knowing about adverse drug reactions (ADRs), deaths caused by the drug or even the types of drugs, good or bad.

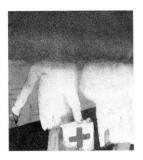

CHAPTER FOUR *WHO WILL BUY?*

D rug companies have been called a two-headed beast. One head could almost be described as cerebral: it's interested in research, and the people it employs are serious-minded academics, usually with first-class science degrees. The other is more reptilian. It's the sales arm that has to claw back the vast amounts spent on researching the newly licensed drug.

As we've seen, the sales team has a window of just a few years when it has exclusive rights to the new drug before its patent lapses. In that time, they must at the very least recoup the research and development costs, which could be up to £350 million.

The first requirement is to create a need for a drug. This might sound strange, but marketing professionals would understand the expression. We don't really 'need' a new car or a new mobile phone, but advertisements associate the acquisition with a better life, a prettier girlfriend or more handsome boyfriend, for instance.

Although drugs are there to ease the symptoms of a recognised disease or condition, they follow the same priniciple. The implicit selling techniques of the drugs industry was made explicit by Fred Nadjarian, managing director of Roche in Australia. In an interview, he revealed how a drug company went about selling a drug. He used for his example the marketing of Roche's antidepressant moclobemide, marketed in the UK as Manerix.

A press release in Australia revealed that one million Australians suffered a "soul-destroying" psychiatric disorder called social phobia. What the Australian public didn't know was that Roche had sponsored the publicity and that they were about to launch moclobemide, specifically designed to treat 'social phobia'.

Nadjarian suspected he had been a victim of his overzealous marketing department when Roche tried to recruit some of the million sufferers for a trial of the drug. Quite simply, the patients weren't out there.

Social phobia is a disease affecting very few people, if any, in fact. Nadjarian points out that the example of social phobia is true for a wide range of diseases. "If you added up all the statistics, we all must have about 20 diseases. A lot of these things are blown out of all proportion," he said.

While drug companies sponsor press publicity, academics are also keen to exaggerate the prevalence of a disease as it can draw attention to their own research. "Behind every statistic there is a vested interest," said Nadjarian.

His comments add weight to a growing belief that the practice of exaggerating the prevalence and seriousness of a disease is widespread in the pharmaceutical industry (BMJ, 2002; 324: 867).

The vast majority of new drugs are 'me-too' in the sense that they offer a variation on an existing drug that might be doing a similar job. That being the case, how do you convince a doctor to switch to your drug, which has had very limited safety trials, and stop using a drug that at least is tried and tested?

In the UK, there is a code of practice that forbids any inducement to encourage a doctor to prescribe a drug. For instance, Clause 18 states: "No gift, benefit in kind or pecuniary advantage shall be offered or given as an inducement to prescribe, supply, administer, recommend or buy any medicine except certain, inexpensive promotional aids and competition prizes that are relevant to the recipient's work."

There is, however, a useful loophole in Clause 19 which

allows for "appropriate hospitality . . . such as scientific and promotional meetings, provided the hospitality is secondary to the main purpose of the meeting".

So, stories about inducements of computers and cash are a thing of the past. Or are they? In Germany, for instance, authorities there have just uncovered a giant bribery web that involved over 100 hospitals. Some doctors had been handed cars, computers and paid-for trips, while others had accepted cash payments of up to £15,000, from employees of SmithKline Beecham. The scandal, which involved thousands of doctors, has attracted a great deal of interest, not least from the German wing of Transparency International, the anticorruption group. A spokeswoman said: "This is a normal practice in the drug industry. Our organisation has done a lot of research on bribery and corruption in the German health sector in the past three years, but the pharmaceutical industry has not changed its habits" (Lancet, 2002; 359: 1039).

In the USA alone, drug companies spend around $2 billion a year on events for doctors, so exercising full use of the Clause 19 loophole. This can include dinners and 'conventions' where the ostensible reason to attend is to learn something about a condition—although the sponsoring drug company will have a drug that happens to treat that condition—and doctors are usually handed a cheque of between $500 and $2,000 for turning up.

Any doctor who is uneasy about accepting what, after all, is a blatant bribe might be prepared, instead, to participate in a trial after the drug has been awarded its licence.

The final requirement under the Medicines Act is for the drug to undergo a post-marketing surveillance study to monitor side effects. This area has been subject to the greatest abuse, and has been described by Dr Bill Inman, who set up the Drug Safety Research Unit, an independent monitoring agency of drug reactions, as marketing dressed up as research. Patients unwittingly have been switched from a safer, effective course of treatment to a new drug so that the doctor can claim his gift or financial reward.

Amounts earned vary; Dr Vernon Coleman, a critic of conventional medicine, reckons doctors can earn an additional £50,000 a year by prescribing the new drugs to large numbers of patients; the British Medical Association says the agreed sum per report is £7, although there can be 10 Yellow Card reports per patient. "I blew the whistle on one product where a doctor had 230 patients in a study for rheumatoid arthritis when he had only five sufferers in his practice. He alone was responsible for 10 per cent of the entire market for that drug," said Dr Inman. He carried out a survey among 28,402 GPs in Britain and discovered that just 10 per cent of GPs are responsible for creating 42 per cent of a new drug's total market, so putting at risk their patients when the drug's side effects are not properly known (BMJ, 11 September 1993).

A report by the Medicines Control Agency in 1992 revealed that 31 post-marketing trials were inadequate, biased and poorly designed (BMJ, 1992; 204: 1470–2). In America, the FDA has set up MedWatch to encourage health professionals to report side effects. Currently, it estimates that only 1 per cent of side effects are reported to the FDA (JAMA, 2 June 1993).

One of Dr Inman's greatest successes, achieved shortly before he retired in 1993, was to have included in a code of practice to all doctors the stipulation that no treatment should be changed just so that a patient can be included in a study of a new drug. Nonetheless, it is just a guideline with no compulsion to adhere to it and, in reality, it is mostly ignored.

The most scandalous aspect of the post-marketing study is that the drug company is not obligated to publish the research; it must inform the drugs authorities but, under Section 118, it need not reveal these data to the public. This means that a drug company and a drug authority can be aware of a serious side effect, even though a GP is still prescribing it. He, of course, would be as ignorant of the findings as the patient.

Fortunately, in two recent cases, the pharmaceutical company acted responsibly when further tests showed a possible side effect not picked up by the limited clinical trials. In April 1993, Boots withdrew its 100 mg Manoplax tablets, licensed the previous September to treat congestive heart failure. Tests in the US, Canada and Scandinavia found that patients were more likely to die of heart failure with the drug than without it. About 900 patients received the drug at the more dangerous dosage level. In June 1992, the antibiotic Teflox was withdrawn in the UK after

20,000 patients had been given it in just eight months. The US manufacturer Abbott Laboratories discovered that the drug could cause liver and kidney problems, and a life-threatening shock reaction. Section 118 of the Medicines Act has also prevented an explanation of why the tranquilliser Halcion was withdrawn at 24 hours notice in 1991, or why two of the three vaccines for the measles–mumps–rubella (MMR) shot were withdrawn after a £20 million government promotion.

It sometimes happens that only when side effects are reported by the media, or discovered by an independent research group, that the dangers of a drug become known. For example, nobody knows how many people a year die as a direct result of drugs. Global figures are released by the Committee on Safety of Medicines, but they are not itemised to specific drugs. For instance, it revealed that 280 people died from taking prescribed drugs in 1987, yet the Medical Research Council estimates that 600 people die each year in the UK from taking non-steroidal anti-inflammatory drugs (NSAIDs) alone. However, Professor Michael Rawlins, a former chairman of the CSM, estimates that only 10 per cent of all serious adverse reactions are ever reported to the authority. Drugs expert Dr Joe Collier has estimated that 100 people could die if a new drug with an unknown, lethal adverse reaction were prescribed to 30,000 patients.

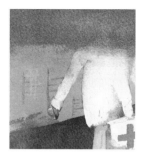

CHAPTER FIVE *THE RESEARCH GOES ON*

The drug has been licensed for use, it's been through the early post-marketing surveillance study and it's getting some way towards recouping the £350 million investment in it. It's also been supported by a marketing campaign that has again raised the ante.

But that's not it for the drugs company. It has to keep the pot boiling to both reassure doctors that they have made the right decision in prescribing the drug and to attract other doctors who may be influenced more by proper, scientific trials than by a free lunch.

The findings of the trials are often published in one of the prestigious medical journals, such as The Lancet, the New England Journal of Medicine, the Journal of the American Medical Association or the British Medical Journal. The trials will often involve large numbers of people who will be taking the drug, and the results of the therapy will be matched against a similar-sized group called the 'control'.

The drug company itself will often pay for the research, although independent researchers, usually from a university or a research hospital, carry it out. As it is pure research, the researchers should be presenting their findings as they discover them, without interference from the paymaster.

Although the study will often run to five or six pages in one of the journals, most people read just the summary at the beginning, which sets out the objectives of the study, the numbers involved and the findings.

That, anyway, is the theory. The fact that we are a long way from that has been highlighted by a joint statement, prepared by the editors of 12 of the world's leading medical journals, including the ones mentioned earlier, that states they are no longer prepared to publish studies ". . . where the author of the study can't state that they had access to the entire data and an entirely free hand in writing it," said John Hooey, editor of the Canadian Medical Association Journal.

The statement is the culmination of years of concern about fraudulent research and findings that may have been tampered with by the drug companies.

Although this is a practice that has been going on for years, the extent of the interference came to light in a battle between a researcher, Dr Nancy Olivieri, a haematologist at Toronto's Hospital for Sick Children, and the Canadian drug company Apotex Inc. The company hired Dr Olivieri to conduct trials of deferiprone, their new drug for patients with the inherited blood disorder thalassaemia. The drug company cut her research grant after she published a critical article about the possible adverse reactions of the drug, which included liver damage.

This is but one of many examples. A British pharmaceutical fraud investigator reckons that fraud takes place in between 1 and 5 per cent of all medical trials. This may not sound much, but at least 3,000 sponsored clinical projects take place in the UK at any one time—which means that between 30 and 150 of them are presenting false data.

The investigator, Medico Legal Investigations, said examples of fraud included a surgeon who said he had assessed a patient who, in fact, had died six months earlier, while another doctor was said to be assessing blood flow in the leg of a patient that had already been amputated! Another doctor forged 191 patient signatures and other data in 21 studies.

Fraudulent research and incomplete data have been reported, and even the British Medical Journal has published a book on the subject, *Fraud and Misconduct in Medical Research* (BMJ

Publishing Group, 1993). The FDA has discovered "serious deficiencies" in 11 per cent of clinical trials in the US. In the UK, the antiarthritis drug Opren had only one clinical trial among the over-65s, and no tests were done to assess how different doses work in different age groups. Despite this, a licence was granted in the UK, whereas the FDA waited for further tests. Over 4,000 Britons, many elderly, contacted the Opren Action Group alleging some injury, mainly an increased and persistent sensitivity to light, and a further 100 were reported to have died.

Deficiency is one thing, fraud another. While the level of fraud in clinical trials is not known in the UK, it is reckoned that "a small but significant amount of data . . . is fraudulent," according to Dr Frank Wells, medical director of the Association of the British Pharmaceutical Industry (ABPI). However, medical critic Dr Vernon Coleman states: "It is now reliably estimated that at least 12 per cent of scientific research is fraudulent" ('Betrayal of trust', Eur Med J, 1994).

Similar stories have come out of the USA. There, findings are sometimes exaggerated to make a drug sound better than it really is, while positive findings tend to be published in several different journals—usually changing the names of the researchers involved—to give the impression that these are new studies.

Needless to say, company-funded research tends to favour company products. For example, a 1998 report in the New England Journal of Medicine revealed that 96 per cent of authors of research papers whose research was favourable to some heart drugs had financial ties to the drugs' manufacturers.

A study published in the Annals of Internal Medicine revealed that 98 per cent of company-sponsored drug studies published between 1980 and 1989 in journals made a positive conclusion about the funding company's drug.

Drug companies often own and control the data collected in trials they have sponsored. This means they can filter the data to the researchers who have to analyse it. So, for instance, some poor results can be lost or mislaid, and only the most positive outcomes are released for further analysis.

More recently, the American Heart Association accepted an $11 million donation from drug company Genentech while it was preparing practice guidelines on stroke management. By the time the report was published, Genentech's thrombolytic drug was recommended in the guidelines.

Overall, it's reckoned that 70 per cent of all medical research is underwritten by the pharmaceutical industry (N Engl J Med, 2000; 342: 1539–44). Researchers are being asked to sign confidentiality agreements before beginning the research, which effectively gags them from speaking out if anything fraudulent or 'unscientific' should happen during the research or analytical process.

It's hard for researchers to fight back. One who did ended up with a $10 million lawsuit against him and his university after he insisted on publishing research into a drug company's AIDS vaccine that found the drug to be of little benefit.

Sometimes, researchers are paid for their research. Sometimes, if your name is prestigious enough, you will be paid for putting your name to research you've never seen. Ghostwriting is now widespread in areas such as cardiology and psychiatry, where drugs play a major part in treatment.

One author's ties to a drug company were so involved that the New England Journal of Medicine could only find sufficient space for them on its website. "Researchers serve as consultants to companies whose products they are studying, join advisory boards and speakers' bureaux, enter into patent and royalty arrangements, agree to be the listed authors of articles ghostwritten by interested companies, promote drugs and devices at company-sponsored symposiums, and allow themselves to be plied with expensive gifts and trips to luxurious settings. Many also have equity interest in the company," wrote Marcia Angell, former editor of the New England Journal of Medicine.

Sometimes, 'independent' books on an illness, and the drugs to treat it, are prepared for health professionals. These books take the form of ongoing training, and are usually handed out free to thousands of doctors and consultants.

So who pays for this beneficence? Drug companies, of course. They are the unseen hand that guides the editorial that might conclude that a particular drug, which happens to be manufactured by the sponsoring company, coincidentally turns out to be the best available on the market.

Normally, this subtle form of marketing goes on undetected. Unfortunately, it came seriously wrong for one drug company recently. The company paid for the book by way of an "unrestricted educational grant", and the editors came up with the conclusion that the company's drug was ideal as an immunosuppressant following liver transplant.

Unfortunately, they were overzealous in their efforts to please their sponsor. In the few trials undertaken, patients who had taken the favoured drug after a liver transplant had died within 30 days.

In fact, the drug company had pulled its drug from further trials, so embarrassed were they by earlier findings.

The influence of the drug companies goes further than just academic books. It is reckoned that up to one-third of all MPs in the British Parliament receive some funding from a drug company to help pay for administrative expenses and the like.

Journalists are 'retained' by drug companies so they can wax lyrical about a new drug or some promising research. This latter ploy is a particularly favourite for the Sunday newspapers that seem to fill their columns with stories of exciting breakthroughs and cures that, strangely, are never heard of again. It's done wonders for the drug company's share price, nonetheless, as stock markets live more in hope than on solid, hard fact.

One study into the media's coverage of drugs found that the mainstream press and broadcasting outlets never spoke about the side effects of drugs, or the financial ties that 'independent' researchers had with the manufacturer. The study team looked at 207 newspapers and TV stories from 1994 to 1998, and their coverage of three drugs that were in the news during that period: aspirin; Zocor, a cholesterol-lowering drug; and Fosamax, an osteoporosis drug.

In the 170 stories that cited experts or scientific studies, half included at least one expert or study that had financial ties to the drug company concerned. Fewer than half the stories talked about the drugs' side effects (N Engl J Med, 2000; 342: 1668–71).

Drug companies also like to make donations to charities that represent a specific disease. That way, no alternative remedy gets to see the light of day, and the donor's particular drug tends to be mentioned more often than that of its competitor.

In most cases, we are talking about relatively small sums of money, but it is enough to buy subtle influence, and ensure that the lid is kept tightly on a scandal that would otherwise blow apart the world's most profitable industry.

In summarising the state of affairs in medicine today, an editorial in the Lancet asked: "How tainted by commercial conflicts has medicine become? Heavily, and damagingly so, is the answer" (Lancet, 2002; 359: 1167).

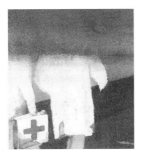

CHAPTER SIX *GUINEA PIGS ARE WE*

S tudies and trials are one thing; the real test of any drug—new or old—takes place 'in the field', where it is prescribed every day to thousands of people who unwittingly take part in the greatest experiment of them all, usually with their health, and sometimes their lives, at stake.

Around one in five drugs will have a serious side effect 'discovered' after all the expensive licensing procedures and trials have been completed. Sometimes, the effect can take up to 25 years to uncover, as revealed by a study from Harvard Medical School (JAMA, 2002; 287: 2215–20).

The researchers monitored the progress of 548 new drugs that were approved for use in the American market between 1975 and 1999. They checked to see if they were either withdrawn, or went on to receive a 'black-box warning' in the American drugs bible, the *Physicians' Desk Reference*. The black-box warning appears at the very beginning of the description of the drug, and alerts the medical professional to a very serious adverse reaction that is usually life-threatening.

It's important to note that the Harvard researchers restricted themselves to the very serious adverse reactions that would result either in death or permanent disability. The more common side effects discovered after the drug was licensed, but which can also ruin a person's life, were not even included in their research.

Of the 548 drugs tracked, 56, or 10.2 per cent, acquired a new black-box warning—which means a very serious side effect was discovered only when patients started taking the drug—or were withdrawn altogether because the potential side effects were so serious that they were probably a threat to life.

In addition, another 45 drugs, or 8.2 per cent, acquired one or more black-box warnings, and 16 were withdrawn from the market.

Overall, the likelihood of a new drug acquiring a new black-box warning or of being withdrawn from the market was 20 per cent. Half of the changes happened within seven years of the drug reaching the market, and half of all withdrawals occurred within the first two years.

However, this means that half of all the deadly drugs were not detected quickly, so exposing millions of people to a dangerous drug. The longest time it took to give a drug a new black-box

Drugs taking the longest time to receive a new black-box warning		
Drug	**Warning**	**Time taken (yrs)**
Pemoline	liver toxicity	22.9
Disopyramide phosphate	**increased risk of death**	**19.3**
Ketoconazole	heart complications	15.6
Danazol	**strokes**	**15.5**
Cyclosporin	hypertension	14.2
Captopril	**unsafe during pregnancy**	**11.7**
Mitozantrone	bone marrow toxicity	10.0
Propafenone	**increased risk of death**	**9.2**
Ribavirin	increase in artery pressure	8.0

warning was nearly 23 years in the case of pemoline, a central nervous system stimulant, which was finally discovered to cause liver poisoning (see box for worst cases).

The time to withdraw a drug from the market was usually much swifter, but then, drug regulators were dealing with reactions that often resulted in death. While some drugs were withdrawn within months of their introduction, some went on for years before finally being removed.

The worst example found by the Harvard researchers was terfenadine, an antihistamine that had been prescribed for nearly 13 years before it was discovered that it could cause serious heart problems if the patient was taking another drug at the time.

Similarly, astemizole, another antihistamine, reacted badly with other drugs, but this was not discovered for nearly 11 years.

The drugs industry is riddled with examples of drugs which have serious side effects that are not discovered until they are prescribed *en masse* to the public; in fact, that is exactly how side effects are discovered.

The class of cholesterol-lowering drugs known as statins, to take one example, was thought to have very few side effects. However, as doctors started prescribing them in numbers, they found that male patients were complaining that they had suddenly become impotent. This would usually happen within a week of starting treatment. Doctors at Guy's Hospital in London discovered the problem when five male patients reported the side effect to them (how many more kept quiet is anybody's guess)— but how could they be sure the drug was the culprit?

When the doctors turned to the datasheets, which are the official documents released with the drug and are based on the early marketing trials, they could find no mention of impotence as a possible side effect. It was only when they delved deeper and looked at the findings of the Australian Adverse Drug Reactions Committee that they found the answer. The Australian committee had received 42 reports from men complaining of impotence after taking simvastatin, one of the statins. The problem had often occurred within 48 hours of starting treatment (BMJ, 1997; 315: 31).

This is an object lesson that highlights several of the central problems. It shows the inadequacies of the early trials that determine whether a drug should be approved and, but for the perserverence of the doctors at Guy's, impotence may never have been recognised as an adverse reaction to a statin. How many times has a doctor not recognised a reaction because it was not already listed and so, instead, blamed the reaction on some other aspect of the patient's life rather than on the drug itself?

Sometimes a reaction may be far more serious than temporary impotence. Sometimes patients die before a drug is withdrawn, as happened with Lotronex (alosetron), a drug to treat irritable bowel syndrome (IBS) in women.

The drug was approved for use in America by the drug regulator, the Food and Drug Administration (FDA), on the basis of two 12-week trials that involved 1,273 women. Overall, the drug was far more effective than a placebo (sugar pill), against which it was tested.

However, researchers had noted that four cases of colitis were reported during the trials, but each case was short-lasting, mild and reversible once the drug treatment was stopped.

But soon after the drug was approved in February 2000, the FDA started receiving reports of more serious reactions of intestinal damage and ruptured bowels. The first cases were received within weeks of the approval being granted and, by November, the FDA had 70 cases of serious 'adverse events', including three deaths.

It's interesting to note that even faced with this overwhelming evidence, the FDA did not withdraw the drug's licence. The drug's manufacturer, however, decided to withdraw the drug from the market as the possibility of lawsuits started to loom.

Lotronex had a shelf life of just nine months before it was withdrawn from the market. Others, which have caused far more suffering, have lasted longer. Take, for example, the case of Prepulsid (or cisapride, its generic name), which was designed to treat heartburn. It was finally withdrawn from the UK market in July 2000, four months after the FDA announced that 80 people in the USA, and a further 10 in Canada, had died as a result of the drug.

This four-month interval is alarming enough, but the Committee on Safety of Medicines, the UK drugs watchdog, said that reports had been coming in of fatalities since the drug won its licence in 1988, 12 years before it was finally withdrawn.

Nobody knows for sure how many people died while on the drug, but conservative estimates put it at around 125, plus a further 50 suspicious deaths. In addition, there had been 341 cases of serious heart rhythm abnormalities reported in the USA, 44 in Canada and 60 in the UK.

Drugs seem to be getting more toxic. Since 1997, more drugs have been proven toxic and been withdrawn than in any other era in the history of modern medicine. Some of the withdrawn drugs were prescribed millions of times before the authorities acted. Dr Alastair Wood, from the Vanderbilt University Medical Center in America, reckons 19.8 million patients—which equates to 10 per cent of the US population—have been exposed to just five of 10 drugs withdrawn since 1997.

Sadly, Dr Wood added, "None of the drugs was indicated for a life-threatening condition nor, in many cases, were they the only drugs available for that indication" (JAMA, 1999; 281: 1753–4).

Britain and the USA are not two isolated, albeit significant, examples. Dr Thiery Buclin, a Swiss health official, has said that, in 1998 alone, of the 30 medicines approved that year, five had to be removed later. He puts the blame squarely on the prelicensing process, which he believes can be too hasty, and then on the post-licensing period, when drugs are aggressively marketed. "We have proof of too much hastiness and sometimes a lack of prudence. The pharmaceutical industry plays the first role in this dangerous game. With aggressive marketing, it uses heavy infantry to convince health personnel" (from an interview in *Dimanche* newspaper, 2 April 2000).

Even death can sometimes not be enough to get a drug removed from the market. After Viagra, the impotence drug, had been on the market for seven months, the FDA reported receiving 230 cases of deaths associated with the drug. But this did not result in the withdrawal of the drug; instead, the FDA insisted the manufacturer change the warning on the label.

Only the drug regulators themselves can explain why they were so slow to react to drugs such as Prepulsid and others like them that endanger people's lives and wellbeing, but as they are not accountable to the public, there is no way of knowing.

The meetings of the UK's Committee on Safety of Medicines are held in secret, and minutes from those meetings are not made available to the public. Indeed, every meeting begins with a reminder to all those present that the proceedings are secret and cannot be discussed with anyone outside of the room.

Experts from drug companies fill many important, and

influential, positions on various advisory groups. More than half the experts sitting on committees of the FDA have financial relationships with the pharmaceutical industry.

If, as is the case, every new drug is an experiment, what can the practitioner—and you, the patient—do? The most obvious solution, as suggested by the Harvard researchers at the conclusion of their study, is to avoid all new drugs if a proven alternative is already available on the market.

This is clearly the sensible approach but, as we have seen in earlier chapters, it is not the way the drug industry works. They are under enormous and continual pressure to produce new drugs. The cost of this process can be astronomical, and so it is much more cost-effective to produce a 'me-too' drug rather than a groundbreaking one. Even so, the licensing process for a 'me-too' drug can still be expensive and lengthy, giving the salesforce a very limited window of opportunity to recoup the investment before the drug passes out of patent.

In short, the Harvard recommendation will never be taken up by the industry.

The licensing process is also geared in such a way that it is not in the drug company's interests to carry out exhaustive trials before a licence is awarded. By the time the drug reaches the premarketing stage, the drug company has already spent a good part of the £350 million average investment on the new drug. It hardly wants to uncover nasty side effects at that late stage and so, as the Harvard researchers point out, the early trials are "often underpowered to detect ADRs (adverse reactions), and have limited follow-up".

Most drugs are prescribed to the elderly, but the elderly are rarely involved in any of these early trials. The elderly may also be taking a cocktail of drugs, and nobody ever investigates the possible interactions between them. Many serious adverse reactions are, in fact, a result of the interaction between the different chemical compounds of the variety of drugs being taken, as we shall see in the next chapter.

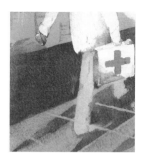

CHAPTER SEVEN *WOMEN AND CHILDREN FIRST*

To understand the enormous gulf that lies between the data collected from the premarketing trials and the information that is discovered once the drug is prescribed, we have to remind ourselves who takes the drugs.

Drugs are, by definition, taken by people who are 'ill'; this means that you have a range of symptoms that medicine feels are worthy of treatment.

A woman passing through the menopause may not be ill, but she has symptoms that have launched the single most lucrative area of drug sales, hormone replacement therapy (HRT). A younger woman who does not want to become pregnant is not ill, but she wants a contraceptive pill. Similarly, a young child who is deemed to be hyperactive (ADHD) may not be ill in the conventional sense, but again fits the Identikit for treatment with Ritalin or one of the other amphetamines.

It's interesting to note that some of the most profitable drugs do not treat illness at all, but could instead be described as 'lifestyle' drugs.

Add the over-50s to these groups and you have the three main groupings of prescription drug usage in the West: young children, menopausal women and people over the age of 50.

So, how representative are the premarketing trials that

determine if a drug is safe for use? Are they packed out with young children, menopausal women and older people?

In the UK, ethics committees—usually created within the drug company undertaking the trial—insist that neither children nor women "of childbearing potential" should be recruited to participate in trials, and certainly not in the early stages of a drug's development. Mysteriously, those who are responsible for recruiting volunteers must also ensure that the participants are healthy, so presumably people who are ill are excluded.

Although children are rarely, if ever, part of the early marketing trials, there is a wide range of drugs aimed at them. It's almost as if the drugs industry has adapted the old Jesuit maxim 'Give me the child, and I'll give you the man' to 'Give me the child, and we've got a customer hooked for life'.

In America, it's been reckoned that over 3 billion prescriptions are filled out every year, which equates to every man, woman and child in America receiving one prescription every month of the year.

The most common family of drugs prescribed for children is the antibiotics; it's been estimated that antibiotic prescriptions represent over a third of all prescriptions written for children. Many are inappropriately prescribed as antibiotics are effective only against bacterial infections, and not virus-related diseases.

Although they are among the most common drugs, they can still cause serious side effects. Anaphylactic, or allergic, reactions strike with varying degrees of intensity in up to 10 per cent of patients, and the reaction can be fatal in 1 in 50,000 cases. Other reactions include anaemia and seizures, while overuse can result in infestation of the gut as well as resistance to antibiotic treatment later in life.

Ritalin and other amphetamines have been described as drugs in search of a disease. They are now the first-line treatment for hyperactivity, or ADHD, or ADD, a convenient tag for a wide range of symptoms that could merely indicate the natural, restless energy found in many young children.

Dubious though ADHD may be as a genuine condition, Ritalin has been so overprescribed in the USA that the World Health Organization has issued a warning against its overuse.

The European Commission recently urged pharmaceutical

companies to devote more resources to develop drugs specifically for children. This would mean that more accurate dosages could be given, and pills could be better designed for swallowing by small mouths and throats.

The EC recognises that up to 90 per cent of all licensed drugs have never been evaluated for use by children—so confirming that children do not participate in premarketing trials—and yet they are prescribed for children once approval has been granted.

Serious errors in calculating the correct dosage for children can lead to serious adverse reactions, the EC believes, so drug companies are being asked to develop and research drugs with children specifically in mind.

To sweeten the pill—as if drug companies needed any incentives to open a new and lucrative market—the EC is considering granting much longer patents to give a drug company a greater monopoly once a licence has been granted. It is also considering the creation of a special fund to help pay for such research. Europe is following the lead of the USA where over 400 drug trials involving children have already been held in the last few years (BMJ, 2002: 324: 563).

Another lucrative market has been menopausal women. To convince women that the menopause is a disease was perhaps the single greatest marketing coup by the drug companies in the 1990s. As a result, the HRT drug Premarin became the single most prescribed drug ever; in 1999 alone in America, 47 million prescriptions were written. Premarin is like the veal of the drugs industry; the way it is made—from the urine of mares kept locked in very restrictive stables—has incensed animal rights groups.

This clearly has not put off too many women nor has the range of side effects that fills three pages of the *Physicians' Desk Reference*, the American drugs bible. The direst warnings concern increased risks of developing endometrial cancer with this oestrogen-only preparation, a danger which has been shown in three independent studies. The risk can increase by nearly 14 times if the drug is taken for more than one year. Other side effects include cancer of the breast, cervix, vagina and liver (as shown in animal studies), gallbladder disease, heart attack, stroke, high blood pressure, bleeding, nausea, headaches and weight gain, to name but a few.

Most drugs are, however, reserved for the elderly (certainly those aged considerably beyond the over-50s definition given earlier). Over one-third of all prescriptions are made out to elderly patients, who are usually already taking multiple prescriptions to treat a range of disorders.

One study of the medical records of 283 elderly patients found that 11 per cent of visits to a hospital accident & emergency unit were related to a complication caused by a drug. The study found that, on average, patients were taking four drugs, while 13 per cent were taking up to eight different drugs (Ann Emerg Med, 2001; 38: 666–71).

It is this combination-cocktail effect that can produce serious, if not lethal, reactions, as a later chapter will explore.

The prescribing of drugs to the elderly brings into the sharpest focus all the problems of drug licensing and marketing that have been outlined in earlier chapters. A study by the US Department of Health and Human Services concluded, "A major factor in the number of adverse drug reactions among the elderly is their doctors' over-reliance on promotional materials provided by the drug manufacturers" (Drug Safety, 1991; 4: 247–65).

Drug companies are often at pains to claim that their new drug is well tolerated among the over-65s. They say this because they know this is where the major part of their market is to be found. But, as we have seen, how do they know this when the elderly have been excluded from trials to evaluate the safety of the drug?

Even without the cocktail effect, individual drugs are quite capable of doing harm without the aid of any compatriots. This is because the changes in the older body means a drug is metabolised differently. Reduced blood flow in the gastrointestinal tract makes the absorption of drugs slower, as does decreased body weight.

So, again, we return to the question: If the elderly, who are the main recipients of drugs, metabolise drugs differently from younger people, why are they not recruited more into prelicensing trials?

The answer is simple, of course. If you've got £350 million riding on the successful outcome to a drug trial, the last thing you want is elderly people reacting badly to it, and so delaying or even preventing its approval.

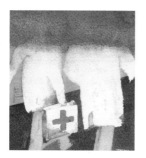

CHAPTER EIGHT *TOO MANY DRUGS...*

Y ou have a mild heart condition, joint pains and a cough—
a not unlikely trio of complaints. But go to your doctor
and you could easily find yourself on the receiving end
of 16 different drugs—two for your heart (perhaps aspirin and
digitalis), a third one for arthritis and a fourth to counter the side
effects of the third; you then pop along to the chemist for a cough
remedy which itself might contain a dozen different compounds.
You're now deep in drug-interaction territory, a no-man's land of
medical Russian roulette.

Because so much of modern conventional medicine is based
on drugs, and doctors (and some patients) have been led to
believe that there's a pill for every ill, it's hardly surprising that
more and more people are taking more than one medication at a
time.

Multidrug-taking, or polypharmacy as it's known in the trade,
is obviously not discouraged by the pharmaceutical industry, but
there is growing concern within some of the more enlightened
parts of the medical profession of the potential for hazardous
interactions between drugs.

An American report showed that the side effects and
misprescribing of medications result in "drug-induced disorders"
of epidemic proportions, costing the US economy a staggering

$136 billion a year—quite apart from the toll in human suffering and even death. The authors point out that ". . . many adverse drug events occur as a result of drug–drug or drug–food interactions, and therefore, are preventable" (Am Fam Physician, 1998; 57: 2615–6).

Detailed studies have revealed the potential scale of the interaction problem. Researchers at the University of Southern California Medical Center showed that the risk of an adverse drug interaction rises from 13 per cent for patients taking two medications at the same time to 82 per cent for patients taking seven or more (Am J Emerg Med, 1996; 14: 447–50).

Exactly how many people experience drug interactions is not known. Figures vary widely, but a review of the records of over 370,000 patients showed that up to 70 per cent may have been affected by adverse drug–drug effects (DICP, 1990; 24: 982–9).

That drug companies should wish to develop drugs that require long-term use makes commercial sense, and they are constantly on the lookout for new chronic conditions to treat. Drugs have even been developed for people who aren't ill and have no true symptoms, such as 'patients' with high blood pressure or high cholesterol.

Often, the side effects of drugs don't become apparent for years and, when they do, doctors are not discouraged from continuing the drugs, but often prescribe yet more drugs (dubbed 'chasers' by some industry insiders) to counteract the side effects of the first. This polypharmacy is, of course, highly profitable. Sometimes, however, doctors won't even be aware they're prescribing a chaser drug.

"There is no doubt that the unwanted effects of a drug are not recognised as drug side effects, and therefore a new diagnosis is entered into and a new drug prescribed," admits clinical pharmacologist Professor Patrick Vallance of University College London.

However, polypharmacy is routinely used for many chronic conditions, such as heart disease and arthritis.

Medications for heart disease and high blood pressure abound—there are ACE inhibitors, calcium antagonists, anticoagulants, antiarrhythmia drugs, alpha-blockers, beta-blockers, stimulants and diuretics—and cardiologists claim that combining them can often produce a beneficial additive effect. But, with the co-administration of so many drugs, there is a danger of overloading the body's ability to metabolise them and causing kidney failure, particularly in the susceptible patient (Drug Safety, 1995; 12: 334–47).

Interactions are particularly a problem when one of the drugs has a critical dosage, such as the heart drug digoxin—too little won't work, too much may be toxic. If other drugs interfere with the absorption and metabolism of digoxin, the side effects may poison the patient.

Amidst the welter of heart drugs, cardiologists themselves have questioned what is 'rational' polypharmacy and what is not (J Hum Hypertens, 1991; 5: 9–14). To add to the confusion, chaser drugs have now been developed to counter the side effects of digoxin.

But it's in arthritis therapy that chaser drugs have reached their apogee.

The major treatments used in arthritis are the so-called non-steroidal anti-inflammatory drugs (NSAIDs). Most of the major drug companies have products in this area: brand names include Advil, Aleve, Anaprox, Ansaid, Clinoril, Feldene, Lodine, Motrin, Naprosyn, Nuprin, Relafen and Voltarol. Many of these are related to aspirin, but are chemically different enough to allow them to be patented and sold at a higher price. However, despite their apparent sophistication, NSAIDs exact an equally high price on the patient, for they often cause serious stomach ulceration. In fact, a recent study by Professor Michael Langman of the University of Birmingham has shown that NSAIDs are responsible for up to a quarter of all cases of, and a quarter of all deaths from, peptic ulcer bleeding (Ital J Gastroenterol Hepatol, 1999; 31: S2–5). In the US, an estimated 70,000 people are hospitalised annually because of the ulcers caused by NSAIDs (J Musculoskeletal Med, 1991; 8: 21–8).

To counter the side effects of NSAIDs, at first, doctors used cheap, non-prescription antacids, but the drug companies soon weighed in with two patented antiulcer 'improvements'—Zantac (ranitidine) and Tagamet (cimetidine). Sales rocketed and these two drugs are now among the most successful in the history of the pharmaceutical industry.

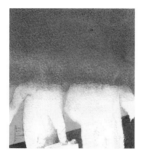

CHAPTER NINE *LET'S ADD CHEMICALS*

W hy are drugs so dangerous? Part of the problem is, as we have seen, their interaction with each other. But another reason could well be their added ingredients—the additives, or excipients as the drug industry calls them. These additives are supposed to make the drugs look and taste appealing, maintain their shelf life and help the active ingredients blend together properly.

More than 700 chemical agents are used as excipients in drug products (N Engl J Med, 1983; 309: 439–41), but only a few have been fully researched to determine their safety. Because these compounds are classified as 'inactive', there are no regulations requiring listing them on product labels. Many excipients, such as flavourings and fragrances, even fall under the heading of 'trade secrets', so manufacturers are exempt from full disclosure of these chemicals on their labels.

Adverse reactions to drugs are common. Patients reporting such reactions to drugs are often not taken seriously because doctors can find no link between the symptom and the active ingredient. Yet, some inactive ingredients have a major role to play in adverse drug reactions.

These chemicals are known to cause a number of health problems, including allergic reactions (Can Med Assoc J, 1984;

131: 1449–52; Med Toxicol, 1988; 3: 128–65; 209–40). One review went so far as to declare that "excipients should not be considered as inactive ingredients as they have been associated with a wide range of adverse reactions in some individuals" (Drug Safety, 1990; 5 [Suppl 1]: 95–100).

The more problematic excipients include certain preservatives, sweeteners, solvents and dyes known to cause a variety of symptoms—from respiratory difficulties to headache, skin rashes, gastrointestinal upsets and diarrhoea, as well as less obvious reactions such as hyperosmolality (an increased permeability of body cells and tissues allowing the exchange of otherwise separately contained fluids).

Preservatives

A variety of antimicrobials and antioxidants are added to drugs to prolong shelf life and maintain sterility. The most commonly used antimicrobials include chlorbutol, benzyl alcohol, sodium benzoate, sorbic acid, phenol, thimerosal, parabens and benzalkonium chloride. Common antioxidants include butylated hydroxytoluene and hydroxyanisole as well as propyl gallate and sulphites (Med Toxicol, 1988; 3: 128–65; 209–40).

While necessary to ensure the safety of pharmaceutical products, the inclusion of preservatives has also been associated with a range of adverse effects.

Benzyl alcohol, for example, can cause several hypersensitivity reactions. Contact dermatitis (Contact Derm, 1975; 1: 281–4) as well as more general allergic reactions such as nausea, fatigue, fever, maculopapular rash or angioedema (localised water retention in the blood vessels) have occurred after parenteral administration of products preserved with benzyl alcohol (Acta Allergol, 1958; 12: 295–8; N Engl J Med, 1982; 306: 108).

The link between benzyl alcohol and neonatal cardiovascular collapse—dubbed 'gasping baby syndrome'—is perhaps the most widely publicised adverse reaction related to 'inactive' ingredients. The relationship was discovered in 1982 after a series of newborns died or developed a severe respiratory illness associated with gasping, metabolic acidosis (an overly acidic body pH) and blood abnormalities.

Eventually, the cause of this syndrome was determined to be intravenous flush solutions and medications containing benzyl alcohol (N Engl J Med, 1982; 307: 1384–8; Am J Perinatol, 1984; 1: 288–92). As a result, both the US Food and Drug Administration (FDA) and American Academy of Pediatrics recommended that, whenever possible, infants should avoid products containing this chemical (MMWR, 1982; 31: 290–1; Pediatrics, 1983; 72: 356–8).

The incidence of premature infant mortality, severe neurological symptoms and intraventricular haemorrhage decreased significantly after discontinuation of the use of benzyl alcohol in intravenous drugs intended for infants (Pediatrics, 1986; 77: 500–6; Pediatrics, 1989; 83: 153–60).

While not all infants exposed to this chemical died, many of those who survived suffered from one of a range of illnesses associated with exposure, including cerebral palsy and developmental delay (Pediatrics, 1986; 77: 507–12).

But it's not just infants who react badly to benzyl alcohol. In one report, a man who used a nasal spray containing albuterol diluted in a solution of benzyl alcohol reacted with severe bronchitis and blood-stained sputum (JAMA, 1990; 264: 35).

In older patients, benzyl alcohol continues to be associated with a range of hypersensitivity reactions such as contact dermatitis, nausea, bronchitis and a range of adverse neurological events (Contact Derm, 1999; 41: 302–3; Am J Contact Derm, 1999; 10: 228–32; J Fam Pract, 1995; 40: 35–40; Med J Aust, 2000; 173: 141–3).

Another common antimicrobial, benzalkonium chloride, has received considerable attention over the past several years as a result of its use in many nasal sprays and metered-dose inhalers (it is also found in numerous 'natural' products, most recently, grapefruit seed extract). In some asthmatic patients, benzalkonium chloride can produce significant respiratory distress.

In a study by Zhang and colleagues of 28 asthmatics, a significant decrease in lung function—which began within a minute and lasted up to 60 minutes—was observed after benzalkonium chloride administration (Am Rev Respir Dis, 1990; 141: 1405–8). The authors noted that the response was blocked by the simultaneous administration of the antihistamine cromolyn, suggesting an allergic mechanism.

In non-asthmatic patients, the use of nasal sprays with benzalkonium chloride has been associated with burning, dryness and irritation of the nasal passages (J Allergy Clin Immunol, 2000; 105: 39–44). It has also been linked to increasing nasal congestion. Inclusion of this chemical explains, in part, the rebound congestion seen with prolonged use of such products (Clin Exp Allergy, 1994; 25: 401–5; Clin Ther, 1999; 21: 1749–55).

Flavourings

A wide variety of natural and synthetic flavourings are used in the production of pharmaceutical products. In a survey of oral medications, Kumar and colleagues (Pediatrics, 1993; 91: 927–33) found that more than 90 per cent of the products they evaluated contained both sweeteners and flavourings.

In this survey, 35 per cent of the products evaluated did not provide information on flavourings, making it difficult to identify the specific causes of adverse reactions or allergies. Menthol, lemon oil and peppermint oil have all been associated with hypersensitivity reactions in children.

Few, if any, manufacturers fully disclose what goes into their flavourings, preferring to hide behind the labelling loophole of 'trade secret'. Yet, flavourings contain numerous ingredients. For example, one brand of synthetic strawberry flavouring contained more than 30 different components (Neurosci Biobehav Rev, 1993; 17: 313–45).

Sugar-free, but not risk-free

In addition to flavourings, a variety of sweeteners are used in drugs. Saccharin, sucrose, sorbitol, aspartame and fructose are the most commonly used sweeteners and, often, two or more of these are present in oral liquid preparations.

The concentration of sweeteners in oral solutions and suspensions ranges from 30 to 50 per cent of the formulation. In some antibiotic and cough/cold preparations, the sweetener content can be as high as 80 per cent (Am J Hosp Pharm, 1988; 45: 135–42).

As sucrose in oral medicines has been shown to result in an increased risk of tooth decay in children (Pediatrics, 1981; 68: 416–9; Public Health, 1994; 108: 121–30), the current trend is towards the use of artificial sweeteners, such as aspartame and saccharin.

But the use of artificial sweeteners brings its own problems. Aspartame, an excitotoxin (a central nervous system stimulator), is increasingly being used in chewable tablets and sugar-free formulations of drugs and supplements.

Headache is the most common adverse effect linked to aspartame. Up to 11 per cent of patients with chronic migraines report that their headaches are triggered by aspartame (Headache, 1989; 29: 90–2). This effect, however, has been disputed in the medical press. In one double-blind, placebo-controlled trial, for example, three doses of aspartame given every two hours to patients who believed their migraines were made worse by aspartame triggered no more headaches than did placebo (N Engl J Med, 1987; 317: 1181–5). However, a small, double-blind four-week trial showed an increase in frequency of headaches after ingestion of 1200 mg daily of aspartame, suggesting that it may take longer for adverse reactions to become apparent (Headache, 1988; 28: 10–4). Other studies have also confirmed the aspartame/headache link (Neurology, 1994; 44: 1787–93).

In anecdotal reports, aspartame has been linked to conditions such as panic attacks, mood changes, visual hallucinations, manic episodes and isolated dizziness (Lancet, 1986; *ii*: 631; Lancet, 1985; *ii*: 1060; Psychosomatics, 1986; 27: 218, 220; Am J Otolaryngol, 1992; 13: 438–42). A small, double-blind, crossover study of patients with major depression found that these individuals may be more sensitive to the effects of aspartame than non-depressed subjects. Taking 30 mg/kg of aspartame for seven days resulted in a higher incidence of adverse reactions, including headache, nervousness, dizziness, impaired memory, nausea, temper outbursts and depression (Biol Psychiatry, 1993; 34: 13–7).

In the US, passive surveillance data collected by the FDA showed a link between seizures and aspartame consumption (Lancet, 1985; *ii*: 1060; Psychosomatics, 1986; 27: 218, 220; Neurology, 1993; 43: 2154–5). This finding, however, was disputed by a randomised, double-blind, placebo-controlled trial (Epilepsia, 1995; 36: 270–5).

Nevertheless, though aspartame is generally considered safe for children with epilepsy, one study found increased spike-wave discharges in children with untreated absence seizures after a high dose of aspartame. The authors also suggested that children with poorly controlled absence seizures should avoid the sweetener (Neurology, 1992; 42: 1000–3).

A few hypersensitivity reactions resulting from ingestion of aspartame have been reported, including two patients who developed inflamed bumpy skin resembling erythema (Ann Intern Med, 1985; 102: 206–7; J Am Acad Dermatol, 1991; 24: 298–300). Other reported reactions include orofacial granulomatosis (inflammation of the skin around the mouth), erythema, pruritus (itching), urticaria (hives) and angioedema (vascular water retention) (Am J Clin Nutr, 1986; 43: 464–9).

Such reactions are thought to be rare (J Allergy Clin Immunol, 1991; 87: 821–7; J Allergy Clin Immunol, 1993; 92: 513–20) and, some argue, may not be necessarily related to aspartame *per se*. Instead, they may be related to breakdown products such as diketopiperazine derivatives, formed during the storage of liquid products, especially after exposure to higher temperatures (Ann Intern Med, 1986; 104: 207–8).

If this is the case, it may explain why challenging sensitive individuals with fresh aspartame powder sometimes produces false-negative results (the subject is sensitive, but the results indicated no sensitivity). Although not yet fully researched, there is a possibility that aspartame breaks down into the carcinogen formaldehyde, as suggested in some animal experiments (Life Sci, 1998; 63: 337–49).

Saccharin

Another common sweetener, saccharin can be present in substantial amounts in drugs. A sulphonamide derivative, saccharin can cause skin reactions similar to those associated with other 'sulpha' drugs. Studies have demonstrated cross-sensitivity with sulphonamides; therefore, those with a sulpha allergy should also avoid saccharin.

In 42 patients who had adverse effects due to consumption of saccharin in pharmaceutical agents, itching and hives were the most common reactions, followed by eczema, photosensitivity and prurigo (a blistering, crusting rash) (NZ Med J, 1989; 102: 24). Other reported reactions included wheezing, nausea, diarrhoea, tongue blisters, rapid heart rate, headache, diuresis (excessive urination) and sensory neuropathy (nerve pain) (J Allergy Clin Immunol, 1974; 53: 240–2; J Allergy Clin Immunol, 1975; 56: 78–9; Cutis, 1972; 10: 77–81; J Am Acad Dermatol, 1986; 15: 1304–5).

A major large-scale FDA/National Cancer Institute (NCI) epidemiological study concluded that ingestion of the recommended daily dosage of chewable aspirin or acetaminophen (paracetamol) tablets in a school-age child would provide roughly the same amount of saccharin as a can of a diet soft drink. Prolonged periods of ingestion of this amount, given the body weight of a child aged under 9 or 10 years, is considered "heavy use" (Lancet, 1980; i: 837–40). In this study, heavy use of artificial sweeteners was associated with a significantly increased risk for bladder cancer.

An independent review of this study, however, refuted this finding (Am J Public Health, 1982; 72: 376–81). A later animal investigation of saccharin by the American Medical Association concluded that bladder changes were species-specific (confined to the second generation of male rats), and occurred in association with large doses (equivalent to several hundreds of cans of diet soft drink a day) (JAMA, 1985; 254: 2622–4).

Nevertheless, many agencies, including the US Environmental Protection Agency (EPA) and National Academy of Sciences, concluded that, even though human data are lacking, saccharin should still be considered a potential human carcinogen.

Lactose

Although a sugar, lactose (milk sugar) is more widely used as a filler or diluting agent in tablets and capsules, and to give bulk to powders. Although most people can tolerate this sugar without adverse effects, some experience hypersensitivity reactions. Those who are lactose-intolerant have been reported to develop diarrhoea even with the intake of the small quantities found in tablets.

Sensitivity to lactose varies widely in severity, although some (adults and children) may experience diarrhoea, gas or cramping after ingestion of as little as 3 g or less of lactose (Am J Clin Nutr, 1972; 25: 467–9; Gastroenterology, 1973; 65: 735–43). Such symptoms have been noted in sensitive persons after taking drugs containing lactose (N Engl J Med, 1978; 299: 314; N Engl J Med, 1986; 315: 1613–4; J Clin Psychiatry, 1992; 53: 328–9). There have been two reports of adult asthmatics who developed bronchospasm from lactose-containing medications, and who tested positive in double-blind challenges with 300 mg and 500 mg of lactose (J Allergy Clin Immunol, 1976; 57: 440–8; Eur J Respir Dis, 1984; 65: 468–72).

Lactose can also cause complications in those with lactase deficiency. This condition occurs either as a rare congenital disorder or is acquired in later life. Its symptoms include diarrhoea, abdominal cramping, bloating and flatulence after ingesting milk products or lactose.

Late-onset lactase deficiency (adult hypolactasia) is surprisingly common. Around 90 per cent of adult American blacks, 60–80 per cent of Mexican Americans, Native Americans and Asians, and most Middle Eastern and Mediterranean populations have abnormal findings on lactose tolerance tests (Am J Dig Dis, 1973; 18: 595–611; Am J Clin Nutr, 1972; 25: 869–70; Gastroenterology, 1977; 72: 234–7; Am J Dig Dis, 1971; 16: 1123–6, 203–6). Approximately 10 per cent of the white population of Scandinavian or European ancestry are also affected (N Engl J Med, 1975; 292: 1156–9).

Solvents

Medications that are not highly water-soluble are problematical for pharmaceutical manufacturers. To render the product soluble enough for oral, topical or intravenous use—without significantly altering its stability—a variety of solvents, such as propylene glycol and polyethylene glycol, are used (Med Toxicol, 1988; 3: 128–65).

In particular, propylene glycol—used in topical, oral and injectable medications—has been associated with cardiac arrhythmias, seizures and respiratory depression.

The high concentration of this agent in drugs such as

phenytoin, phenobarbital, diazepam, digoxin and etomidate may induce thrombophlebitis (inflammation of a vein associated with a blood clot) when administered intravenously (Br J Anaesth, 1979; 51: 891–4, 779–83).

For this reason, these medications need to be administered slowly when given intravenously. Rapid infusion of concentrated propylene glycol-containing drugs has been further associated with respiratory depression, cardiac arrhythmias, hypotension and seizures (Am Heart J, 1967; 74: 523–9).

Intravenous solutions containing propylene glycol have also been associated with seizures, and liver and kidney damage (J Child Neurol, 1998; 13 [Suppl 1]: S11–4; Am J Kidney Dis, 1997; 30: 134–9) as well as haemolysis (loss of haemoglobin from red cells), central nervous system depression, hyperosmolality and lactic acidosis (Lancet, 1984; i: 1360; J Anal Toxicol, 1985; 9: 40–2; Arch Intern Med, 1991; 151: 2297–8). Case reports continue to show that intravenous propylene glycol can be toxic (N Engl J Med, 2000; 343: 815; Crit Care Med, 2000; 28: 1631– 4; Am J Crit Care, 1999; 8: 499–506).

Several cases of localised contact dermatitis from the application of products containing propylene glycol have also been reported (Arch Dermatol, 1971; 104: 286–90; Cutis, 1980; 26: 243–4; Contact Derm, 1989; 21: 274–5; Contact Derm, 1985; 12: 33–7). These include propylene glycol-containing jellies, such as those used in electrode placement, and steroid creams (South Med J, 1980; 73: 1667–8; Arch Dermatol, 1979; 115: 1451; Contact Derm, 1979; 5: 53–4).

In 487 patients with eczematous contact dermatitis, 4.5 per cent were found to be sensitive to propylene glycol (J Am Acad Dermatol, 1982; 6: 909–17).

But propylene glycol doesn't have to be applied to the skin to cause skin reactions. Oral and parenteral preparations can also cause dermatitis in sensitised patients (Contact Derm, 1978; 4: 41–5; Semin Dermatol, 1982; 1: 49–57).

Recently, GlaxoWellcome issued a warning against its anti-HIV drug, the protease inhibitor amprenavir (Agenerase), which contained a large amount of propylene glycol. The company revealed that some patients—such as infants, pregnant women, those with kidney or liver problems as well as those treated with disulfiram or metronidazole—were not able to metabolise propylene glycol adequately, leading to its accumulation in the body and a range of adverse effects (Pharmaceutical J, 2000; 264: 685).

Propylene glycol is particularly dangerous in infants. This is because newborns have a longer propylene glycol half-life (16.9 hours) compared with adults (five hours) (JAMA, 1985; 253: 1606–9; Pediatrics, 1983; 72: 353–5).

The propylene glycol contained in an intravenous multivitamin product delivering 3 g/day was associated with a higher incidence of seizures compared with lower doses from an alternative product delivering just 300 mg/day (Pediatrics, 1987; 79: 622–5). In addition, seizures and respiratory depression were seen in children who ingested liquid medications containing propylene glycol (J Pediatr, 1970; 77: 877–8; J Pediatr, 1978; 93: 515–6).

These are just some of the adverse reactions associated with some of the most commonly used excipients. Many more excipients are used, but have never been fully investigated for safety.

Reactions to chemicals such as aspartame and propylene glycol may be even more common because our exposure to them extends beyond mere drug use to the foods we eat, herbal and nutritional supplements, and even toiletries.

Clearly, these 'inactive' ingredients can have a profound effect on health. Until manufacturers are compelled by law to list all of the ingredients in their drug preparations, such reactions will continue to be commonplace.

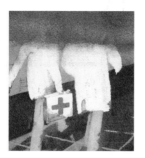

CHAPTER TEN *A DRUG CHECKLIST*

As with medical tests, before you take any drug, it's vital that you learn as much as you can—indeed, more than your doctor—about it. Every drug marketed in the UK has a datasheet, which is essentially a profile of the drug at a glance, listing when it should or shouldn't be taken, and also its side effects. All these datasheets are bound up in a publication called *The Medicines Compendium* (which used to be called *The Data Sheet Compendium*). You can also find out information about drugs from *MIMS*, the drug bible of most doctors (although copies are expensive).

Once you've read up on the drug being proposed for you (and if you have only the one office visit, ask for the data sheet on the drug right then and there), put in following questions to your doctor:

● How long has this drug been on the market? As we have seen, many of the problems of drugs and their side effects come with the newer drugs that have been recently licensed and are being aggressively marketed by the drug company's salesmen. If your doctor takes you off a particular drug and tries another drug that he says will work better, be very suspicious—you may be an unwitting guinea pig in a drugs trial.

● Is drug therapy really needed for this problem? Many

conditions, such as premenstrual tension or depression after a bereavement, can be treated by diet or the loving attention of friends and relatives. A new study finds that people suffering from major depression can be helped just as well by being helped to face up to and solve their problems as by taking antidepressants. Unless you can be persuaded that your condition will definitely worsen, why introduce a substance that could also introduce a whole new set of problems?

- What will happen if I don't take the drug?
- What is this drug supposed to do for me? How will it do that? How are you going to monitor the use of the drug? Do your instructions differ for those of the datasheet?
- What sorts of drugs or substances (including non-prescription drugs, food or alcohol) should I avoid when taking this drug?
- With what other drugs does this drug dangerously react? Although one drug used alone might carry a small risk, when combined with another drug, that risk may be multiplied several times over, as can the strength of the toxicity.
- What are the known side effects of this drug, as reported by the manufacturer? (Don't settle for vague assurances by your doctor; request that he read out loud from *MIMS*, there and then.)
- What are the latest reports in the medical literature about this drug's side effects? Journals like The Lancet publish new studies all the time demonstrating that the risk of a certain drug are far higher than the manufacturer originally thought. If he doesn't know, go to the science reference library in a large city. Most large science libraries will have the US *Physicians' Desk Reference* or *The Medicines Compendium* on the shelf. The British Library's medical section holds both. Another possibility is to do a Medline search, a computerised version of the *Cumulative Index Medicus*, a summary of most scientific studies carried out on most treatments. If your library doesn't have Medline, they probably have the *Index Medicus* itself, unwieldy volumes that will fill most of a shelf. Otherwise, visit a large medical bookshop. Many useful drug books are for sale in general book shops. Your best source for full information about drug side effects is to own your own copy of the *Physicians' Desk Reference*. If you can't get hold

of a copy in Britain, ask your American friends or relations to stuff a *PDR* into their suitcase the next time they come to visit.

- May I discontinue any other drugs I am currently taking? The American Health Research Group suggests that, if you are taking other drugs, have a 'brown-bag session' with your doctor—that is, place all the medications you're taking (including non-prescription drugs) into a carrier bag and bring it to your doctor so that, together, you can determine if any work together synergistically (it also makes sense to do a drug worksheet, so that you don't mix up what you are taking).

- Under what conditions and how should I stop taking this drug if I notice certain side effects? What sorts of tests are available to monitor my reaction to the drug?

- If I don't wish to take this drug, what other possible therapies are there for me to consider? You might need to gently prod your doctor into enumerating the possibilities he's heard of, not offer an opinion. Doctors simply don't believe in non-drug therapies. For one thing, very few of them know anything about it.

If you decide to take the course of drug, become your own laboratory. Look out for any unusual symptoms your body starts displaying. You might suddenly have difficulty sleeping, or may be you start getting dizzy spells. If you start experiencing conditions you've never had before, suspect the drug, and report the effects to your doctor immediately.

Unfortunately, as we have seen, medicine is notoriously bad at reporting adverse reactions and side effects, so you could find yourself in a pharmaceutical Catch-22. If your doctor doesn't see your symptom listed, he may assume the drug cannot be to blame. You might come to the same conclusion if you can't see your newly-acquired symptom among those listed in any of the drug reference books.

If all else fails, contact the American Food and Drug Association. Anyone around the world has the right of access to information about drugs licensed by the FDA, courtesy of the American Freedom of Information Act. Write a letter to the address below asking for the Summary Basis of Approval (SBA) for your drug (make sure to find out the American generic and brand name first, as drug names can differ on either side of the Atlantic). The SBA includes a detailed summary of the data, including results of clinical trials, that formed the FDA's decision to approve the drug. Also ask for Adverse Drug Reactions (ADRs)—unverified reports of any side effects reported—including new MedWatch reports (the new database of drug reactions recently set up by the FDA). Finally, ask for any reviews or assessments of ADRs, which will put these isolated reports of reactions in context. (Bear in mind that American drugs can be licensed in different doses than British ones and for different conditions.)

You will be charged $3 per request; after the first 100 pages of photocopying and first two hours of research, which are free, you are charged 10 cents per page of photocopying and a fee of $13–$46 per hour, depending upon the grade level of the person required to do the research. (In your letter, you can ask for an estimate of how much your search will cost.) Write to:

Food and Drug Administration
Freedom of Information Office
5600 Fishers Lane
Rockville, MD 20857
USA

They must respond within 10 days, if only to say that your request is being investigated.

The Medicines Compendium can be purchased direct from the publishers:

Pharmaceutical Press
P.O. Box 141
Wallingford, Oxon OX10 8QU
(tel: 01491 829 272; fax: 01491 829 292)

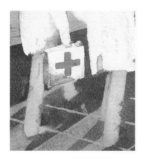

CHAPTER ELEVEN *AND IN THE END*

Every time a patient picks up a prescription from the doctor, he or she is about to embark, unwittingly, on a vast experiment. There is a tacit understanding between the patient and the doctor that the drug being prescribed is relatively safe. At the very least, there is an expectation that the benefits of the drug will far outweigh any possible risks. If a drug can ease excruciating pain and make life bearable, if not comfortable, then the 'price' of feeling a little dizzy sometimes is one worth paying.

Indeed, in the majority of cases, this is precisely the kind of trade-off that does take place, and that is why the scandal of the harm that drugs can do never comes to light. As a society, we accept that drugs are properly monitored and managed, and that their benefits far outweigh any harm they may inadvertently cause.

Such unspoken assumptions underpin much of our everyday lives. We assume that the airplane we are boarding is far more likely to land safely at its destination than crash and kill all the occupants. And our experience supports that. We read about one or two major crashes a year and, when it happens, there is always a thorough review of safety regulations to see if there is a way of ensuring that such an accident never happens again.

Death from a drug is never so dramatic but, regrettably, it is far more frequent. Indeed, the rate of deaths from drug reactions is so great that it has been equated to a jumbo jet crashing every day. Such a risk in air travel would be unacceptable, and nobody would board an airplane again until they had sufficient assurances that all the problems had been resolved, and that it was safe.

By comparison, a drug death involves one person dying quietly in a hospital bed or at home, and he or she was probably quite old anyway. It happens at an alarmingly high rate, as we have seen but, inevitably, it always happens to an individual and an individual death never makes the headlines, not even if it is happening hundreds of times every day around the country.

Not only does it happen quietly, it often goes unrecorded. A doctor rarely reports the fact that the patient died from the drug. This may be because he didn't make the connection himself, or perhaps the current literature doesn't suggest that a fatal reaction is possible, or perhaps the doctor is overwhelmed by the amount of paperwork he already has to complete. Sometimes, the possibility of legal action also plays a part.

A drug often has what is known as a paradoxical effect—in other words, it produces the very symptoms it is supposed to treat. Sometimes, therefore, the illness is blamed as the cause of death rather than the real culprit, the drug itself.

Death is, of course, at the extreme end of the spectrum of adverse reactions. Many more people suffer a serious reaction to the drug, so serious that their lives will never be the same again. It has been estimated that 40 per cent of all drug treatments is ended prematurely because the reactions to the drug are so intolerable that they far outweigh any possible benefits.

Conversely, just 60 per cent of patients see benefits of their drug therapy that outweigh the side effects; this is a slender margin and probably far less than the average citizen would expect. Certainly, a minority of patients suffers more from a drug than benefits from it, but it is a large minority—and if medicine's reporting systems worked properly, may not be a minority at all.

We return to the same question we asked at the outset: why do prescription drugs harm so many people when the licensing procedures all drugs must undergo are so onerous, expensive and lengthy?

We've seen that pharmaceutical companies are the fastest growing, and most profitable, in the world. Their share price, and the excitement generated among shareholders and city analysts, is buoyed by new product. If there is even a whisper that company X might have an answer to disease Y, the share price is likely to soar.

The fact that very few new drugs going through the licensing process are anything more than just 'me-too' copies of existing drugs in the market is neither here nor there. They all get wrapped into the buzz of the next new thing.

Once they have received their coveted licence, the new drugs have around five years left on a patent, taken out 15 years earlier when the research scientist first made his breakthrough discovery in the laboratory, to recoup the average £350 million costs involved in getting the licence, and also to make a profit.

This puts enormous pressure on the salesforce to get the drug prescribed as much as possible, and the only way to do that is by winning the acceptance of the doctor who must act as the drug company's interface with the market—the patient.

But how does the drug company convince a doctor to abandon his prescribing of an existing, and probably established, drug with a relatively proven safety record in favour of a new, untested drug? By holding 'conventions' in exotic locales perhaps, or by paying a doctor for participating in a post-licensing trial, with the patient being the unwitting guinea pig.

The trial that won the drug its initial approval may have involved no more than 1,000 participants; now it is suddenly unleashed on hundreds of thousands of people, mainly elderly and almost certainly already taking a cocktail of other drugs.

It is a recipe for disaster, and that is what happens all too often.

So what of the future? The drugs industry is far too powerful, and successful, to change its ways. As it enjoys margins—the difference between turnover and profit—of around 30 per cent, why should it? As we've seen, the drug regulators—the people who are supposed to represent you and me, and ensure that the drugs we're prescribed are safe—are not accountable to us, and their deliberations take place in secret.

All too often, they seem slow to respond, even when it is proven that a drug is killing people.

Yes, the licensing process is lengthy and expensive, but it is clearly sadly inadequate. The real trial takes place only when the drug is prescribed. And once the drug is on the market, the regulators appear to apply a very light touch.

Not only can we expect things not to change, we can look forward to more of the same, with interest. The European Community is calling on drug companies to start preparing drugs specifically for children. This means that correct dosages, rather than best guesses, can be administered, and the shape of drugs will be altered for easier swallowing by small mouths and throats.

So keen is the EU to see the drug companies respond to their challenge that they are offering taxpayers' money to encourage them—as if the world's most successful industry sector needs encouragement to open up a new, and lucrative, market.

The answer is clear, but unattainable. Drug companies cannot meet the needs of shareholders and work for the benefit of mankind at the same time. There are clearly too many occasions when there is a conflict of interest, and it's the shareholder who will win every time, unless the drug company's hand is forced to do otherwise.

Of all the industry groups, the case for the pharmaceutical industry to be placed in public ownership is overwhelming. Medicine is supposed to be for the public good, not for extraordinary profit-taking. Socialism is now pretty much a dead movement around the world, so the chances of seeing a nationalised pharmaceutical industry are about as great as someone producing a safe drug.

If we can't change the world, what can we do? As an individual, you have the right to ask intelligent questions of your doctor before accepting his prescription. The best, and most obvious, question is simply this: can you tell me how long this drug has been licensed? If the answer is not to your liking (and anything under five years should make you feel very worried), it is reasonable to ask if there is another, similar drug that has been on the market longer.

Even this is no safeguard, but at least it reduces the odds of your receiving a drug with a safety, and efficacy, that has not been properly tested.

I n the first part of this book, we saw how, in general, the drug industry works and why drugs can be dangerous, despite an expensive licensing procedure. We now turn to the particular, and to individual drugs and their side effects.

The material in this part of the book has been taken from the regular Drug of the Month column that has been running in What Doctors Don't Tell You since 1993. In that time, we have reported on over a hundred drugs which have caught our attention for a variety of reasons. Sometimes a reader has asked us to investigate, and sometimes the regulatory authorities on either side of the Atlantic have received reports or even issued a warning notice.

Each of these reports has been thoroughly updated. It's been an interesting exercise because some of the drugs have since been withdrawn when, at the time of writing, we were receiving worrying reports about them.

The tone of the pieces has been, in the main, light because the intention has always been to entertain as well as inform. This should not hide the fact that we are dealing with something very serious that has affected, if not destroyed, many lives. Perhaps the only thing to do as a human is to laugh in the face of death.

Of course, most people don't die from taking most drugs. Many, however, are harmed by taking them and, by that, we mean a significant minority.

We hope you find what follows illuminating; it might even give you the key to a mysterious problem you've lived with, especially if you are already taking a prescribed medication.

Our list is by no means definitive; vast volumes are dedicated to such an enterprise. It might, however, give you a flavour of the problem we may all encounter when a doctor hands us a prescription, and it will hopefully encourage you to do your own research.

It is, after all, your life and your body and, unless you are a Buddhist or Hindu, you probably accept that it's the only one you'll get!

All drugs have the potential to be a problem drug, and statistics suggest that too many are. Here, we look at some of the families of drugs that are known to present some of the greater, and more common, risks.

Asthma drugs

Despite greater diagnostic skills, better identification of causes of the disease and ever-whizzier drug cocktails to treat it, doctors and asthma associations are stymied by the fact that the epidemic incidence of asthma and asthma-related deaths continues to go up. US figures, which analysed data for 1999, showed that the annual death rate due to asthma in people aged between 55 and 64 was 11,297, making it the third major cause of death for that age group after cancer and heart disease.

But these days, it's difficult to determine whether the disease or the 'cure' is responsible for killing off patients. Beta-agonists administered by a metered-dose inhaler, specifically albuterol (salbutamol) and fenoterol, have been associated with an increased risk of death or near death (N Engl J Med, 1992; 326: 501–6). The marked rise in asthma deaths during the 1960s in many countries coincided with the introduction of high-strength isoprenaline inhalers. When the inhalers were withdrawn, mortality fell to previous levels. But the problems haven't just been due to beta$_2$-agonists. In many countries, a rise in asthma deaths occurred in the 1980s, particularly in New Zealand, which two studies showed was linked to the popularity of fenoterol, a type of beta$_2$-agonist, but also of oral steroids and theophylline, another type of asthma drug (Lancet, 1995; 345: 2–3).

Regular inhalation of beta$_2$-agonists has also been shown to cause 'hyper-responsiveness'—that is, excessive constriction of the bronchi—and potentially fatal abnormal heartbeats, or may spread the allergen to more remote airways, thus increasing inflammation, or even cause the bronchial muscles to constrict to a fatal degree.

Over time, these drugs may also make the disease worse. In one study, patients receiving fenoterol four times a day had worse outcomes after six months than those given inhaled drugs only as needed (Lancet, 1990; 336: 1391–6). Regular use of certain beta$_2$-agonists also causes a greater decline in lung function than does 'on-demand' use. And some patients have had symptoms improve once doses of inhaled beta$_2$-agonists were reduced.

Inhalers like Ventolin have many established side effects, including sudden lowering of blood pressure, swelling around the heart and collapse. Allen & Hanburys, the manufacturer of Ventolin, also warns doctors that the drug often has a 'paradoxical effect'—that is, it causes brochospasms, the very condition it is trying to prevent.

Deaths in asthma are often due to the very high doses of drugs from inhalers. In a Canadian study, asthmatics who inhaled 13 or more canisters of fenoterol in a year increased their risk of dying *90 times*. As for salbutamol, those who used 25 or more annual doses in smaller-sized canisters were 40 times more likely to die (Lancet, 1990; 336: 436–7). Although both doses far exceed the recommended limit, asthmatics can grow very dependent on inhalers, reaching for them at the first sign of a shortness of breath.

In fact, the risk of death begins to increase dramatically when only 1.4 canisters a month of inhaled beta-agonists are used, particularly among users of fenoterol. The new long-lasting, high potency beta$_2$-agonists like salmeterol (Serevent), which controls asthma symptoms for 12 hours at a puff, could also exacerbate the problem.

Steroids

After all the bad press for beta$_2$-agonists, many doctors are turning to steroids as a first port of call. Steroids mimic the action of the adrenal glands, the body's most powerful regulator of general metabolism. The discovery of steroids was truly miraculous—a lifesaver for those like the late President John F. Kennedy, who suffered from Addison's disease, or adrenal gland insufficiency.

But, as with antibiotics, what was once reserved for the extreme is now used for the trivial. Steroids are now handed out as readily as antibiotics, even to babies, at the first sign of inflammation. Doctors also maintain a conspiracy of silence about these drugs, pretending that steroids cannot cause the terrible carnage that even the manufacturers admit they are capable of. Steroids routinely cause overactivity of the adrenal glands, which produces Cushing's disease, characterised by a fat abdomen and face, and a 'buffalo hump' on the back of the neck, high blood pressure and muscle weakness. They can also cause muscle wasting, hyperglycaemia, water retention, skin atrophy, bruising and stretch marks, insomnia, serious mood changes, symptoms of schizophrenia or manic depression, osteoporosis, cataracts or glaucoma, menstrual problems, impotence, loss of libido or even allergic shock. There is also the problem of recurrent thrush (*Candida*) of the mouth.

More dangerously, prolonged use of steroids causes the pituitary gland to stop producing ACTH, a hormone which regulates the adrenal glands, needed by the body during stress. Even low doses of inhaled beclomethasone reduce bone formation (Lancet, 6 July 1991). Death due to a lack of adrenal gland function have occurred when patients switched from oral to inhaled steroids without overlapping the drugs.

Doctors also like to pretend that if you inhale or rub on steroids, you are less likely to suffer side effects. But evidence shows that inhaled steroids are not as harmless as medicine supposes. The consensus up to now has been that beclomethasone dipropionate (BDP) of 400–800 mcg daily is appropriate for use in those three to five years of age.

Eczema drugs

With eczema, another illness doctors don't understand, they reach for one or another powerful drug to stamp out the inflammation, but not the problem. The drugs of choice are steroids, the immune-suppressant cyclosporin, or even oral psoralen photochemotherapy (oral PUVA), a treatment option for psoriasis that is linked with genital cancer.

As with inhaled steroids, rub-on steroids have long been touted as the safe alternative to systemic steroids, but there's little evidence to back this up. Increasingly, topical steroids are showing themselves to be every bit as dangerous as their orally delivered cousins. Rub-on corticosteroids can produce an array of serious skin problem, damage organs and cause permanent adrenal suppression. They've also been implicated in Cushing's syndrome in children as soon as a month after treatment and, like the oral variety, may impair the responses of the pituitary and adrenal glands, thus requiring yet more (oral) steroids during illness or trauma.

Like asthmatics, children with eczema are prone to the side effects of the long-term use of steroids, such as stunted growth and adrenal disease. Even hydrocortisone cream, supposedly so mild it is often prescribed for babies, is known to have a myriad side effects, including thinning of the skin especially of the face, stretch marks, delayed healing or ulceration of wounds, suppression of adrenal function and sugar in the urine.

In fact, increasing evidence is emerging to suggest that topical and inhaled steroids can cause the eye damage—cataracts and glaucoma—ordinarily only associated with oral steroids. Cases of psychotic episodes with inhaled steroids, again assumed to be caused only by the swallowed variety, are also coming to light.

Arthritis drugs

With arthritis, medical treatment has an air of desperation. Doctors not only don't know how to sort out the problem, but often make a hash of things throwing a load of potentially lethal drugs at the condition and then prescribing new drugs to deal with the side effects caused by the 'treatment'. Conventional medicine tends to take the view that there is no known cause or cure for arthritis, so all that it can do with certainty is to alleviate your pain.

The most common first-line drug for both rheumatoid arthritis and osteoarthritis used to be aspirin at high doses. This is now virtually replaced by the non-steroidal anti-inflammatory drugs, or NSAIDs, as they're known in the trade. In America, there are at least 14 such drugs on the market; several years ago, one of them (ibuprofen) was taken off the list of prescribed drugs and was made available over the counter. Increasingly, doctors now turn to NSAIDs as a first port of call; in 1984, nearly one in seven Americans was treated with one of these drugs, a figure that is now grossly out of date as they are prescribed for everything from headaches to period pains. Arthritis offers drug companies a $10 billion industry in NSAIDs alone.

These drugs mainly work by inhibiting the synthesis of prostaglandins and, thus, suppress inflammation. (They also do a number of other things, such as interfere with enzyme production, the ramifications of which we don't yet understand.) The problem is that the drugs don't just inhibit the prostaglandin that concerns your joint pain; they roadblock all formation, particularly at such high doses. Since this substance plays a major role in normal gastrointestinal function, NSAIDs, not surprisingly, interfere with it. This can result in gastric erosion, peptic-ulcer formation and perforation, major upper gastrointestinal haemorrhage, inflammation, and changes in the permeability of the intestine and lower bowel (N Engl J Med, 13 June 1991).

Once you begin taking NSAIDs, you multiply by seven times your chances of being hospitalised due to gastrointestinal adverse effects. These statistics could be very conservative; the Food and Drug Administration's own best estimate is that 200,000 cases of gastric bleeding occur each year, with 10,000–20,000 deaths. In the UK, some 4,000 people die each year from taking NSAIDs—double the number of deaths from asthma.

The elderly, or those with a history of peptic ulcers, are at particular risk. The FDA now places a warning with each NSAID prescription: "Serious gastrointestinal toxicity such as bleeding, ulceration and perforation can occur at any time, with or without warning symptoms, in patients treated chronically with NSAID therapy." Because NSAIDs reduce pain, particularly at high doses, they also often mask any indication that something is wrong. For many patients, the first sign that they have an ulcer is a life-threatening complication.

Besides ulcers, even the 'safest' of NSAIDs, ibuprofen, can cause colitis, and indomethacin, naproxen and a sustained-release preparation of ketoprofen may cause perforations of the colon. Because these drugs decrease the mucosal prostaglandins, they may cause a leaky gut, resulting in an increased susceptibility to toxins passing through—a recipe for conditions like colitis.

NSAIDs can also cause blurred or diminished vision, Parkinson's disease, and hair and fingernail loss, and can also damage the liver and kidneys. Doctors from several medical centres, including New York's Beth Israel and Harvard Medical School in Boston, reported seven cases of "significant hepatitis" and one death from diclofenac sodium (Voltaren), although they didn't know whether this drug was any more likely to cause these problems than any of the others.

Hypertension drugs

Hypertension is another area in which a mountainous concoction of drugs rarely does any good against a condition that can usually be cured with judicious diet and exercise. Doctors have ploughed through a variety of drug treatments—diuretics, beta and calcium-channel blockers, reserpine, clonidine, methyldopa—without apparent success. A study of 2,000 patients with high blood pressure from 13 GP practices in England showed that only a little more than half of those taking drugs for hypertension had achieved what is considered even a moderately healthy level (Lancet, 1994; 344: 1019–20). In the US, only a fifth of patients on drugs managed to reach what are considered modest blood pressure goals (less than 140 mmHg systolic and less than 90 mmHg diastolic) set by the US Nutritional and Health Examination Surgery. As for Europe, in a survey of 12,000 patients across five countries, only a third managed to achieve the blood pressure targets set by their doctors (Blood Pressure, 1993; 2: 5–9).

If there isn't much evidence that blood pressure drugs do much good, there's plenty to show they do great harm. One particularly worrisome side effect is hypotension—a sudden drop in blood pressure on standing up—which can cause dizziness and falls. Hypertensive drugs are the major cause of hip fractures among senior citizens. Although all varieties of blood pressure-lowering drugs have been implicated in depression, sexual dysfunction, tiredness and appetite disturbances, diuretics (supposedly the 'safe' blood-pressure drugs) have been shown to cause an 11-fold increase in diabetes, beta-blockers may be behind cancer deaths in elderly men, ACE inhibitors can cause potentially fatal kidney damage or death if given too soon after a heart attack, and calcium antagonists have been linked to severe skin conditions like Stevens–Johnson syndrome. Doctors also use these drugs to treat women with hypertension in pregnancy, even though beta-blockers are thought to adversely effect fetal circulation in pregnancy and ACE inhibitors to damage or kill the developing fetus if given during the second or third trimesters of pregnancy.

Combination heart drugs

Most doctors think that if one drug does some good, then two will double the benefits. The beta-blocker–calcium antagonist combination has become very popular for patients with coronary artery disease. The thinking behind it is that a low dose of the two drugs will decrease the number and severity of attacks of angina (pain around the heart during exertion) better than a high dose of one of the drugs alone, and with fewer side effects. Since many factors influence the balance between the supply of oxygen to the heart and its demands, and a single drug can only counter a few of these factors, doctors have simply assumed that a second heart drug with different chemical actions might work in a complementary fashion. Because drugs for angina often cause rebound circulatory effects, which work against their effectiveness, the other assumption has been that these unwanted effects can be counteracted by a second drug.

However, these two assumptions have never stood up to scientific scrutiny. According to one review of the results of a number of controlled clinical trials, combining a calcium antagonist with a low-dose beta-blocker rarely provides any additional benefits for angina, and can increase adverse reactions by up to 60 per cent.

Epilepsy drugs

With such a spectacular array of drug therapy at their fingertips, doctors aren't particularly good at doing nothing—adopting a wait-and-see attitude to see if a condition clears up by itself. Although doctors these days claim to be more cautious about automatically handing out anticonvulsant drugs to children with mild blackouts and seizures, the conventional wisdom among is still that, unless suppressed by drug treatment, epileptic seizures will recur, and that drug treatment can affect the course of the disease, reducing the risk of early epilepsy turning into an intractable disorder.

The problem is that epilepsy is hopelessly overdiagnosed. Experts at Birmingham Children's Hospital concluded that about half of cases of so-called juvenile epilepsy are wrongly diagnosed. This is significant, as more than half the 340,000 cases of epilepsy in Britain are believed to begin in childhood. Dr Michael Prendergast, consultant child psychiatrist at the Children's Hospital, examined 311 children referred to the hospital with suspected or diagnosed epilepsy and found that 138 of them, or 44 per cent, didn't actually have it. His results are nearly identical to those of a Scottish study completed in 1896 by the Royal Hospital for Sick Children in Glasgow. In that study, Dr John Stephenson, the hospital's consultant paediatric neurologist, found that 47 per cent of the children referred there did not in fact have epilepsy.

It's very difficult to know whether drugs given early make any difference, because untreated epileptics are difficult to find. But those studies that have been performed suggest that drugs make virtually no difference. In one, after 20 years, half the group had gone into 'remission'—a percentage equivalent to that seen in those given drugs. Similar remission rates occurred in a group of patients in Africa and in Ecuador; where treatment was delayed, the six-month remission rates were similar to those of populations given early drug treatment.

Much of the evidence suggests that patients having early treatment with drugs may actually be worse off. In one study, patients with seizures after head injury taking the epilepsy drug phenytoin had more seizures than those taking a placebo. A recent Italian study comparing patients on a drug against those on a sugar pill found that, although the treatment group supposedly had half the risk of a further seizure, thus far, there is no difference between the two groups in terms of remission time.

Doctors really don't have enough information to encourage early treatment with certainty, particularly as all epileptic drug treatments carry a host of potentially lethal effects. In one recent study, side effects were so serious that nearly a quarter of patients on phenobarbitone, and 11 per cent of those on carbamazepine, had to be taken off the drugs. Indeed, all epileptic drugs are potentially lethal; the manufacturer of valproic acid (Epilem in the UK; Depakene or Depakote in the States) warns that patients on the drug have died from liver failure.

Antidepressants

Drug treatment is also highly subject to flavour-of-the-month fads. Once doctors become enthused over a new compound which has seemingly done wonders in one area, they like to try it on every illness that comes along. The latest wonder drug is the selective serotonin reuptake inhibitor (SSRI), or a 5-HT drug, the active compound in Prozac.

One cause (or outcome) of depression and suicidal behaviour is believed to be low levels of the brain chemical serotonin, as happens with lowered cholesterol. Prozac works by increasing the availability of serotonin in the brain by slowing the passage of this neurohormone into nerve cells. Prozac has been sold as an amazing improvement over the older tricyclic anti-depressants because it does not cause sedation, or impair thinking or physical activity, and has fewer side effects for more patients.

Hailed by the media in the late 1980s as the breakthrough for depression we've all been waiting for, Prozac quickly became America's best-selling antidepressant and, after the sellout publication of *Listening to Prozac*, America's best-selling happy pill. Enthusiasts are already planning to widen the use of these types of drugs to include overweight patients, cancer patients experiencing nausea from anticancer drugs, people with obsessive compulsions like handwashing, and even those with postmenstrual syndrome (PMS). And as there is evidence that this kind of drug reduces dependence (unlike Valium and other benzodiazepines) by stimulating the reward mechanism in the brain, doctors are discussing the possibility of using it to help control smoking and dependence on other drugs.

The glossy press about Prozac passes lightly over the more than 100 lawsuits Eli Lilly faces from patients claiming that Prozac led them to suicidal and homicidal thoughts and actions. In one case, a Prozac user killed five people and wounded 12 others at the printing plant where he worked. In another, a woman attacked her mother by biting her, ripping out more than 20 bite-sized pieces of flesh.

Although the US Food and Drug Administration cleared Prozac of this association with violence, medical investigative reporter Gary Null has said that most investigations, including the FDA's, have been anything but impartial; all concerned have had a vested interest in clearing the drug. This view seems to be vindicated by a recent study showing that, of all types of antidepressants, serotonin inhibitors had the highest number of suicides.

According to Eli Lilly's own published warnings on the drug, 10–15 per cent of patients in the initial clinical trials reported anxiety and insomnia, and 9 per cent, particularly underweight patients, reported significant weight loss or anorexia. In one study, 13 per cent of patients on the drug lost more than 5 per cent of their body weight. In other words, 1 in 10 patients experienced the same symptoms from the drug that they were trying to treat.

Prozac has also been known to affect nearly every system of the body, including nervous, digestive, respiratory, cardiovascular, musculoskeletal, urogenital, and the skin and appendages. These side effects include, most commonly, visual disturbances, palpitations, mania/hypomania, tremors, symptoms of flu, cardiac arrhythmia, back pain, rash, sweating, nausea, diarrhoea, abdominal pain and loss of sex drive. Less common effects include antisocial behaviour, double vision, memory loss, cataracts or glaucoma, asthma, arthritis, osteoporosis, stomach bleeding, kidney inflammation and impotence. It also, albeit infrequently, causes "abnormal dreams, agitation, convulsions, delusions and euphoria".

Although it's known as the 'happy drug' by some zealots, Prozac may need a new sobriquet soon with the discovery that it may cause sexual dysfunction in up to a third of users. In an overlooked research paper published in the Journal of Clinical Psychiatry in 1992, F.M. Jacobsen found this sort of level of sexual problems among people taking fluoxetine (the generic name for Prozac). A paper published in the same journal a year later found that the rate of sexual dysfunction while taking the drug was as high as 75 per cent.

Hyperactivity drugs

Ritalin (methylphenidate) is America's other miracle drug, taken by as many as one million American children to control attention-deficit and hyperactivity disorder (ADHD or ADD). Ritalin has been largely resisted by parents in Britain, until media attention recently focused on Ritalin as a drug that can "unlock" a child's potential compared with the supposed limitations of the dietary approach to hyperactivity.

The view espoused by Ritalin promoters is that the drug, an amphetamine, works by correcting biochemical imbalances in the brain. Not only is there no evidence to support such a view, but there is no evidence that Ritalin causes any lasting change. As Ciba, the drug's manufacturer, admits, there are no long-term studies on its safety and effectiveness. Furthermore, *The American Textbook of Psychiatry* shows a 75 per cent improvement with Ritalin compared with a 40 per cent response with a placebo, suggesting that half the response with Ritalin could be purely suggestive.

What we do know is that it suppresses growth, makes a child more prone to seizures and causes visual disturbances, nervousness, insomnia, anorexia and toxic psychosis. It's worth remembering that this drug is a class II controlled substance, like barbiturates, morphine and others with a high potential for addiction or abuse. Uppers supposedly have a paradoxical effect on children, quieting them down but, often, the effects are mixed. Children are subdued during the day, but stimulated at night, unable to sleep.

The entry for the drug in the US *Physicians' Desk Reference* carries a special black-box warning of drug dependence and psychotic episodes:

"Careful supervision is required during drug withdrawal, since severe depression as well as the effects of chronic overactivity can be unmasked." Numerous cases of suicide after drug withdrawal have been reported. One study showed that children treated only with stimulants (rather than drugs and counselling) had higher arrest records and were more likely to be institutionalised (J Am Acad Child Adolesc Psychiatry, 1987; 26: 56–64).

This is a list of the drugs featured in this section according to their type. The listing gives only the product name, not its generic/chemical name.

AIDS DRUGS
Roferon-A
Zovirax
ALZHEIMER'S DISEASE MANAGEMENT
Aricept
ANALGESICS
Aspirin
Tegretol
Vioxx
Zydol
ANTIBIOTICS
Genticin
Rifater
Septrin
ANTIDEPRESSANTS
Dutonin
Efexor
Lustral
Manerix
Prozac
Seroxat
ANTIEPILEPTICS
Epilim
Lamictal
ANTIFUNGALS
Lamisil
Sporanox
ANTIHISTAMINES
Clarityn
Triludan
ANTIMALARIALS
Lariam
Nivaquine
Plaquenil
ANTIPARKINSONIANS
Larodopa
ANTIPSYCHOTICS
Roxiam
ANTIVIRALS
Ciproxin
Relenza

NAME	GENERIC NAME
Accolate	zafirlukast
Adalat	nifedipine
Adifax	dexfenfluramine
Aricept	donepezil hydrochloride
Asacol	mesalazine
Aspirin	aspirin
Baycol	cerivastatin
Becloforte	beclomethasone
Betaferon	interferon beta-1b
Bricanyl	terbutaline sulphate
Brufen	ibuprofen
Burinex	bumetanide
Cardura	doxazosin mesylate
Ciproxin	ciprofloxacin
Clarityn	loratadine
Clomid	clomiphene
Condrotec	naproxen/misoprostol
Cordarone	amiodarone
Cozaar	losartan
Desmospray	desmopressin
Dexedrine	dexamethasone sodium
Didronel	disodium etidronate
Diflucan	fluconazole
Dutonin	nefazodone
Efexor	venlafaxine hydrochloride
Eltroxin	levothyroxine sodium
Emblon	tamoxifen
Epilim	sodium valproate
Evista	raloxifene
Feldene	piroxicam
Fosamax	alendronic acid (alendronate sod
Genticin	gentamicin

NSAID for childhood asthma

calcium antagonist for mild heart conditions

SSRI antidepressant for weight loss

acetylcholinesterase inhibitor for Alzheimer's

aminosalicylate for IBS (colitis)

mild NSAID painkiller

cholesterol-lowering statin

steroid for asthma

'new hope' treatment for multiple sclerosis

asthma drug to stop miscarriage

NSAID for arthritis

diuretic for congestive heart problems

alpha-adrenoceptor blocker for hypertension

antibiotic for anthrax

antihistamine for hayfever

antioestrogen for infertility

NSAID for arthritis

drug for irregular heartbeat (arrhythmia)

angiotensin-II receptor antagonist for hypertension

nasal spray to stop bedwetting

amphetamine for weight loss and ADHD

bisphosphonate for spinal osteoporosis

antifungal for fungal/yeast problems

SSRI-related antidepressant

SSRI-related antidepressant

thyroid hormone for thyroid disorders

oestrogen-receptor antagonist for breast cancer

antiepileptic for epilepsy

non-hormonal treatment for the menopause

NSAID for arthritis

bisphosphonate for postmenopausal osteoporosis

antibiotic for infections

LIST OF DRUGS

81

ASTHMA DRUGS
Becloforte
Bricanyl
Pulmicort
Seretide
Serevent
BLOOD MODIFIERS
PumpHep
Marevan
CANCER DRUGS
Emblon
Megace
CHOLESTEROL-
LOWERING DRUGS
Baycol
Lipostat
Questran
Zocor
DIABETES DRUGS
Rezulin
GASTROINTESTINAL
AGENTS
Asacol
Lotronex
Prepulsid
Phenergan
HEART DRUGS
Adalat
Burinex
Cordarone
Plavix
Posicor
Ticlid
Zestril
HRT & MENOPAUSE
DRUGS
Evista
Livial
Ortho-Gynest
Premarin
HYPERTENSIVES
Cardura
Cozaar
INFERTILITY DRUGS
Clomid
IMMUNO-
SUPPRESSANTS
Imuran
Rapamune
Sandimmun

NAME	GENERIC NAME
Imigran	sumatriptan
Imuran	azathioprine
Lamictal	lamotrigine
Lamisil	terbinafine
Lariam	mefloquine hydrochloride
Larodopa	dopamine
Lipostat	pravastatin sodium
Livial	tibolone
Losec	omeprazole
Lotronex	alosetron hydrochloride
Lustral	sertraline
Manerix	moclobemide
Marevan	warfarin sodium
Megace	megestrol
Minocin	minocycline
Neotigason	acitretin
Nicotinell	nicotine
Nivaquine	chloroquine
Ortho-Gynest	oestriol
Phenergan	promethazine
Plaquenil	hydroxychloroquine sulphate
Plavix	clopidogrel
Pondimin	fenfluramine hydrochloride
Posicor	mibefradil dihydrochloride
Premarin	conjugated oestrogen
Prepulsid	cisapride
Proscar	finasteride
Prozac	fluoxetine
Pulmicort	budesonide
PumpHep	heparin
Questran	cholestyramine
Rapamune	sirolimus

analgesic for migraine headaches

immunosuppressant

antiepileptic for seizures

antifungal

antimalarial

cardiac stimulant for Parkinson's disease

statin to lower cholesterol

oestrogen hormone replacement therapy

proton pump inhibitor for ulcers

for IBS (colitis)

SSRI antidepressant

MAO inhibitor antidepressant

blood-thinning anticoagulant

progestogen for breast cancer

antibiotic for acne

oral retinoid for psoriasis

nicotine patches to stop smoking

antimalarial

topical oestrogen for postmenopause

preoperative and general nausea drug

antimalarial

antistroke therapy

slimming drug

calcium-channel blocker (heart drug)

hormone replacement therapy

motility stimulant for dyspepsia and reflux

antiandrogen for benign prostatic disease

SSRI antidepressant

steroid for childhood asthma

anticoagulant for heart patients

cholesterol-lowering drug

immunosuppressant after organ transplants

MIGRAINE
PREPARATIONS
Imigran
Relpax
MS DRUGS
Betaferon
NSAIDs
Accolate
Brufen
Condrotec
Feldene
OSTEOPOROSIS
TREATMENTS
Didronel
Fosamax
PAEDIATRIC DRUGS
Desmospray
PROSTATE
TREATMENTS
Proscar
PSYCHOTHERAPEUTIC
AGENTS
Dexedrine
Ritalin
Zimovane
SEXUAL
DYSFUNCTION
TREATMENTS
Viagra
SKIN & MUCOUS
MEMBRANE AGENTS
Minocin
Neotigason
Retin-A
Roaccutane
Zorac
SLIMMING & WEIGHT
LOSS TREATMENTS
Adifax
Dexedrine
Pondimin
Xenical
SMOKING AIDS
Nicotinell
THYROID
TREATMENTS
Eltroxin
ULCER DRUGS
Losec
Zantac
Zoton
VAGINAL
PREPARATIONS
Diflucan

NAME	GENERIC NAME
Relenza	zanamivir
Relpax	eletriptan
Retin-A	tretinoin
Rezulin	troglitazone
Rifater	isoniazid
Ritalin	methylphenidate
Roaccutane	isotretinoin
Roferon-A	interferon
Roxiam	remoxipride
Sandimmun	cyclosporin
Septrin	trimethoprim
Seretide	fluticasone propionate
Serevent	salmeterol (xinafoate)
Seroxat	paroxetine
Sporanox	itraconazole
Tegretol	carbamazepine
Ticlid	ticlopidine hydrochloride
Triludan	terfenadine
Viagra	sildenafil
Vioxx	rofecoxib
Xenical	orlistat
Zantac	ranitidine
Zestril	lisinopril
Zimovane	zopiclone
Zocor	simvastatin
Zorac	tazarotene
Zoton	lansoprazole
Zovirax	aciclovir
Zydol	tramadol

antiviral for influenza
analgesic for migraine headache
topical retinoid for acne
antidiabetic for type II diabetes
antituberculous drug for TB
amphetamine for hyperactive children
topical and internal retinoid for acne
powerful anticancer drug
antipsychotic
immunosuppressant for psoriasis
antibacterial
steroid for asthma
beta$_2$-adrenoceptor stimulant for asthma
SSRI antidepressant
antifungal
analgesic for neuralgia
antistroke
antihistamine for hayfever
for impotence
analgesic for arthritis
for weight loss
H$_2$-receptor antagonist for heartburn and ulcers
ACE inhibitor for hypertension and heart failure
for insomnia and anxiety
statin for lowering cholesterol
retinoid for psoriasis
proton pump inhibitor for reflux and heartburn
antiviral for herpes and shingles
opioid analgesic

LIST OF DRUGS

ACCOLATE (zafirlukast)
NSAID for childhood asthma
Zafirlukast (marketed in the US as Accolate) was on course for full UK approval when the US drugs regulator, the Food and Drug Administration (FDA) discovered a possible link between it and a rare and fatal condition called Churg–Strauss syndrome. The warning was issued after six patients on the drug developed the syndrome. The FDA says it "continues to believe that the benefits of this drug outweigh any of its known potential risks". Nonetheless, Zeneca, the manufacturer, is putting a warning on the label, and has alerted doctors throughout the US about the possible association.

The main symptom of Churg–Strauss syndrome is vasculitis, an inflammation of the blood vessels. The small and medium-sized arteries are usually affected, often in the lungs, and the syndrome can itself trigger asthma. Early reactions include flu-like symptoms such as fever, muscle pain, headache and weight loss.

Zafirlukast is a new breed of NSAID (non-steroidal anti-inflammatory drug) which inhibits leukotrienes. These have been implicated in various inflammatory diseases, including asthma, rheumatoid arthritis, allergic rhinitis, psoriasis and inflammatory bowel disease.

The FDA has been quick to say that there is no definite link between the drug and the syndrome as yet. Despite the doubts, the drug is still available in the USA although, for once, the UK drug authorities closed the door to it.

ADALAT (nifedipine)
Heart drug for mild conditions
Nifedipine is a heart drug marketed as Adalat by Bayer in the UK (Miles in the US), and as Procardia and XL by Pfizer in the US. It is used to treat relatively mild heart conditions, such as high blood pressure, and angina chest pain.

According to the American *Physicians' Desk Reference* (*PDR*), nifedipine can bring about a heart attack. "Rarely, patients, particularly those [with severely blocked arteries] have developed well documented increased frequency, duration and/or severity of angina or acute [heart attack] on starting nifedipine or at the time of dosage increase," says the *PDR*. "The mechanism of this effect is not established."

The reason why it can make things worse are not the only things still unknown about this drug. Again, according to the *PDR*, nifedipine has been shown to help relieve angina that is brought on by physical exertion in controlled trials of up to eight weeks duration, "but confirmation of sustained effectiveness and evaluation of long-term safety in these patients are incomplete".

The *PDR* reports that, in trials of over 1,000 patients, other reported side effects included oedema (the abnormal build up of fluid under the skin) in up to a third of patients, plus headache, fatigue, dizziness, constipation and nausea.

Nifedipine can also cause abnormally low blood pressure, and its use should be carefully monitored in patients who are already taking other drugs that may also lower blood pressure.

It can also, rarely, cause congestive heart failure characterised by circulatory congestion and retention of salt and water by the kidneys, particularly in patients taking beta-blockers.

ADIFAX (dexfenfluramine)
Weight loss therapy

Overweight people often dream about a magic bullet that will make them slim overnight. But dexfenfluramine is one bullet that can be hit-or-miss, sometimes with serious consequences.

Dexfenfluramine is a serotonin reuptake inhibitor which makes the patient feel sated. It's available in the US as Redux, marketed by Wyeth Ayerst, and in Britain as Adifax, marketed by Servier.

Not for the first time, the US drug regulators have been far more rigorous than their European counterparts. Its first application was refused by the FDA advisory committee, while the pressure group, Public Citizen's Health Research Group, maintains its risks outweigh any benefits.

The Group says that those on the drug for more than three months are nine times more likely to have primary hypertension of the lung. It also warns that the drug may not be very effective; studies have shown that patients have lost no more than 3.4 kg (about 8 lb) more than those on placebo. The Group advises patients to come off the drug after three months if they have not lost weight in that time, a recommendation that is also voiced by some European regulators.

Common side effects include dry mouth, nausea, constipation, drowsiness, dizziness, headache, mood disturbance, depression, insomnia, nervousness and conjunctivitis.

There's been at least one fatal case of pulmonary hypertension during long-term use of dexfenfluramine, although a direct link with the drug hasn't been established.

A study in 1994 involving animals showed that the drug can lead to persistent and permanent brain damage.

Oh well, there's always dieting, we suppose.

ARICEPT (donepezil hydrochloride)
Alzheimer's treatment
"Mum has Alzheimer's," chirrups an advertisement for the drug donepezil hydrochloride in the medical press, "but she knew I was calling today.' Unfortunately, that's about as good as it's going to get for the visiting daughter.

Although donepezil appears to improve cognitive function in patients with mild-to-moderate Alzheimer's disease, it was not able to improve day-to-day functioning or quality of life as measured by the standard tests when it was analysed in a 12-week, double-blind, placebo-controlled study (Dementia, 1996; 7: 293–303).

The Drugs and Therapeutics Bulletin takes the manufacturer, Eisai-Pfizer to task for basing too many claims on one piece of research. "It is not acceptable to ask doctors to make decisions on the basis of the results of a single, clinically inconclusive trial," its report concludes (Drugs Ther Bull 1997; 10: 75–6).

The Bulletin says it cannot recommend the drug to physicians because the benefits to patients are unclear.

A follow-on study, which analysed the longer-term effects of donepezil over a two-year period, has been published only as an abstract, a partial—and unsatisfactory—way of reporting. A second trial of the drug, involving 450 patients, has also been published only as an abstract.

Standard dosage is 5 mg daily taken just before going to bed. The drug can be prescribed only by a specialist able to diagnose and treat Alzheimer's dementia.

Side effects include diarrhoea, nausea and vomiting, muscle cramps, fatigue and insomnia, which are twice as common while on the drug compared with placebo.

At the moment, there is little to offer an Alzheimer's patient other than supportive care, so any therapy that can offer help is to be welcomed. Donepezil has yet to prove conclusively that it is offering that ray of hope.

ASACOL (mesalazine)
Therapy for IBS (colitis)
Mesalazine, marketed as Asacol, is widely used for inflammatory bowel disease (colitis). This anti-inflammatory is a possible cause of major kidney

problems. The drug was reported 104 times in the UK to the Committee on Safety of Medicines, the drugs monitoring body, for causing kidney and urinary tract reactions.

These included interstitial nephritis (kidney inflammation), which was reported 35 times, nephrotic syndrome (low blood protein and fluid in the tissues) and even kidney failure.

Even so, researchers at the Kent and Canterbury Hospitals fear that adverse reactions to the drug are being underreported by doctors. They estimate that patients taking the drug are five times more likely to develop nephritis, but it may not occur until several months after starting treatment, which explains why doctors are not making the association. The longer diagnosis is delayed, the less chance there is of completely reversing the damage. They estimate that only one-third of cases can be reversed if a diagnosis is not made within 18 months.

Other reactions include headaches and gut problems such as nausea, abdominal pain and diarrhoea, and it can even exacerbate colitis. Early reports also suggest it can cause a lowered blood cell count, and inflammation of the pancreas and the liver.

When it was launched, it was marketed as the drug for colitis with fewer side effects. This was because the manufacturer, SmithKline Beecham, had used just mesalazine, supposedly the safer part of sulphasalazine used in other anticolitis drugs, when preparing the new drug.

Perhaps a fresh look at the marketing stance may be in order.

ASPIRIN
Mild painkiller
An aspirin a day is supposed to keep the heart attack away, and without any nasty side effects.

Doctors have been recommending that people take a mini-dose of aspirin, around 75 mg, as part of their daily regimen, along with walking the dog, putting out the rubbish and getting in late for work.

Over the long term, around 20 years or so, this little discipline should greatly reduce the risk of heart problems in later life, and the dose is small enough not to cause any adverse reactions.

Or so they thought. Researchers know that even moderate doses of aspirin can affect kidney function in some way, but now there are concerns that even small doses could have similar effects.

A study in Israel of 49 elderly patients found that even a three-week course, let alone a 20-year one, was affecting kidney function. After one week of taking the 75-mg dose, average serum uric acid increased by 6 per cent and average uric acid clearance decreased by 23 per cent, both described as "significant changes". These levels did not fully stabilise until a week after the course was stopped (Arthritis Rheum, 2000; 43: 103–8).

Just in case you've not been paying attention over the past decade, aspirin can also cause Reye's syndrome, a potentially fatal inflammation of the brain in children and, more commonly, upper abdominal discomfort, allergic hypersensitivity in asthmatics, and gastrointestinal irritation and indigestion, including bleeding and inflammation of the stomach. Gastric haemorrhage has also been reported. Regular aspirin-takers therefore increase their chances of haemorrhage after an operation such as a tonsillectomy or circumcision, and during labour.

So, if you can avoid having an operation, or conversion to Islam or Judaism, or having a baby for around 20 years, you might just reduce your risk of heart problems.

BAYCOL (cerivastatin)
A statin for cholesterol-lowering
Statins used for lowering cholesterol are reckoned to be some of the safest prescription drugs around. But evidence from the USA suggests that this may no longer be the case.

Doctors have discovered a link between one of the statins—Baycol (cerivastatin)—and muscle weakness, or rhabdomyolysis. Fatal attacks have been noted among elderly patients, particularly with high doses or if they have also been taking gemfibrozil, another cholesterol-lowering drug.

As a result, Bayer, the manufacturer, has withdrawn Baycol from the American market. This final act followed a letter from Bayer sent to doctors and other healthcare professionals that stressed the importance of starting the prescription at a moderate 0.4-mg dose.

Bayer first issued a warning about the possible interaction with gemfibrozil in 1999, so the fact that patients have died since then as a result of the prescribing of the two drugs together suggests that doctors are not reading these alerts. Bayer has also warned doctors to be on the lookout for similar reactions among patients taking other statins, so it will be interesting to see if there is any response to this request.

Even without muscular weakness, Baycol comes with a wide enough array of possible side effects. These include leg pain, water retention, muscle pain, insomnia and sinusitis. Interestingly, a number of muscle-related effects had been noted before the drug was withdrawn.

Rhabdomyolysis was already a recognised side effect, as was muscle cramps. Rhabdomyolysis was considered a rare occurrence, however, and was usually associated with acute liver failure. One of the few warnings about the drug was that it could be dangerous to give to any patient who had a liver complaint.

BECLOFORTE (beclomethasone)
A steroid for asthma
Beclomethasone, the generic name for a range of inhaled corticosteroids used to control asthma, can cause cataracts, researchers have discovered.

They found that users were almost twice as likely to develop posterior subcapsular cataracts as nonusers; while the chances of developing nuclear cataracts were around 50 per cent greater.

The research, carried out among 3,654 people, aged between 49 and 97, from the Blue Mountain region of Australia, found that the risk increased with the duration of treatment and size of the dose; the group at highest risk was those with a lifetime dose of 2,000 mg (N Engl J Med, 1997; 377: 8–14).

Some doctors have been surprised by the findings. The Blue Mountain study is the first to indicate a link between the drug and cataracts, and says that the doses tested in the study are far higher than a normal asthma patient would require.

Nonetheless, the drug has been associated with conjunctivitis in earlier studies, although the most common reaction is headache, which can be experienced by up to a third of all users. The next most common reaction is pharyngitis (throat infection and inflammation) and coughing. Others include nasal burning, pain, muscle pain and tinnitus (ringing in the ears).

But the major worry is for asthma patients who switch from a systemically active corticosteroid to some of the aerosol corticosteroids. Some have died from adrenal insufficiency caused by the change. Other problems have included localised infections by *Candida albicans*.

The Blue Mountain research team says their findings are based mainly on beclomethasone, as this was more readily available at the time. The other popular inhaled corticosteroid, budesonide, would also have produced similar results if it had been tested for long enough, they say.

BETAFERON (interferon beta-1b)
'New hope' treatment for MS
Betaferon (Betaseron in the US) is the great drug hope for multiple sclerosis. It's been hailed as ushering in "a new era in the management of MS".

Little wonder, then, that it was chosen as one of the first drugs to be approved by the new European Agency for Medicines Evaluation (EAME), which grants licences for marketing a drug throughout the EC.

Those of you hoping EAME would be a tougher regulator than the UK's Medicines Control Agency might consider the following. The drug was approved after the European Public Assessment Report confirmed that "the application contains adequate clinical trial data to support clinical safety and efficacy".

Their conclusion contains two questionable statements: "adequate clinical trial data" actually amounts to one study, while the reassuring remark about the "safety and efficacy" of the drug may have raised a few eyebrows in the US. There, one study concluded that the drug can cause suicidal tendencies in patients. One patient committed suicide, while another four tried, among 372 MS sufferers given the drug over three years. These fears have also been voiced in the UK by doctors, even though researchers have said the suicides were linked to the illness rather than the drug. Strange, then, that none of the MS sufferers in the US trial not given the drug ever attempted to take their own lives.

Other adverse reactions can include depression and, in non-MS patients, flu-like symptoms, anxiety, menstrual problems and hypertension have all been reported.

MS sufferers may feel the drug is not as risk-free as they've been led to believe; for the rest of us, we should be warned that the new EC drug regulator may not be quite the watchdog we all may think we deserve.

BRICANYL (terbutaline sulphate)
Asthma drug to stop miscarriage

Who reads drug warnings? Not doctors, it seems. Doctors and obstetricians in particular have been giving pregnant women injections of Bricanyl (terbutaline sulphate) to help them go to full term. Along the way, at least one woman has died, and many others have suffered complications such as chest pains, tachycardia (rapid heart rate), dyspnoea (breathlessness) and pulmonary oedema (water on the lungs).

So serious has the problem become that, in the USA, the Food and Drug Administration (FDA) has issued a warning, telling physicians to stop prescribing the drug for preterm labour.

As the drug is solely intended for treating asthma, the warning sounds reasonable. Apparently, manufacturer Hoechst Marion Roussel has made this clear in information sheets in the American *Physicians' Desk Reference*. But doctors in the UK who wish to continue this dangerous practice need look no further than *The Medicines Compendium* (previously *The Data Sheet Compendium*), where the drug is still recommended for the management of premature labour.

Nonetheless, for US doctors, the practice represents a serious misuse of a drug, and one that is indefensible. Read the small print? These doctors are missing the capital letters!

Bricanyl is a beta-agonist drug designed to relieve acute and chronic obstructive lung disease and to improve lung flow rates. Within five minutes, a 0.25-mg dose has been shown to produce a measurable improvement in flow rates.

But even when it is prescribed appropriately, Bricanyl still offers a range of side effects for the unsuspecting patient. The most frequent, and typical for a drug in its class, are tremor and nervousness; these are particularly common in doses above the normal 0.25-mg dose. Other reported reactions include an increased heart rate, palpitations, dizziness, headache, drowsiness, vomiting, nausea, sweating and muscle cramps.

BRUFEN (ibuprofen)
NSAID for arthritis

Ibuprofen, the generic name of one of the most common of the non-steroidal anti-inflammatory drugs (NSAIDs), is also considered to be one of the less potent. This is not saying much for a family of antiarthritis drugs that accounts for 4,000 deaths.

Despite being supposedly less powerful, ibuprofen has been linked to deaths among asthmatics, and has also caused severe stomach bleeding which has also been fatal, according to the *Physicians' Desk Reference*.

One of the most successful products to contain ibuprofen is Motrin, which is manufactured by Upjohn. Dosages tend to be high because doctors see it as a less powerful NSAID, and the manufacturer says that the daily dosage can reach 3,200 g.

However, doses lower than this have caused serious reactions in the very young and the elderly. One 19-month-old child became unconscious after taking between seven and 10 Motrin tablets, and could respond only to painful stimuli, but recovered four hours later. Elderly patients, for whom the drug is primarily designed, can suffer loss of memory and other cognitive faculties while on the drug. Ibuprofen should not be given to pregnant women.

Other high-risk groups include those with a history of liver, kidney or

LIST OF DRUGS

heart problems as the drug has been shown to exacerbate these conditions.

Common side effects include gastrointestinal problems, reported in up to 16 per cent in one controlled trial, which also found nausea, heartburn, diarrhoea, cramps and vomiting. Other effects, reported in between 1 and 3 per cent of users, include dizziness, headaches, skin rash, tinnitus, oedema (fluid retention) and allergies.

One side effect less noticed, and rarely monitored, is blurred and diminished vision, brought to our attention by a WDDTY subscriber. When this occurs, the drug should be stopped immediately.

BURINEX (bumetanide)
Diuretic for congestive heart problems
Our health officials luxuriate in the idea that we have freedom of information about medicine. Patients are now properly informed, and every door is open. Unfortunately, the reality remains rather different, as one of our readers can testify. She is taking 1 mg of bumetanide daily to treat her heart condition. She has heard that it can attack the bone marrow in 1 in 50,000 people taking the drug. But is this so and, if it is, what is the level of risk? As she points out, when the bone marrow is weakened, even a simple cold can kill.

Finding the answer is not as simple as our administrators claim. "Freedom of information to us is non-existent; the manufacturers will tell the doctors, but not us, and our GPs are run off their feet," she states. Doctors and consultants have a couple of minutes to spare on each patient before going on to the next.

Bumetanide is a powerful diuretic usually given to treat congestive heart failure, or kidney or liver disease. This means that a patient needs to be carefully monitored to ensure that he or she does not become dehydrated, and that water and electrolyte depletion does not endanger the life of the patient.

Common adverse reactions include muscle cramps, dizziness, hypotension, headache and nausea. Other reactions have included vertigo, chest pain, ear discomfort, fatigue, sweating, hyperventilation, dry mouth, upset stomach, renal failure and diarrhoea, most of which could be signs of dehydration.

Turning to our reader's concerns, tests have shown that calcium levels have been affected in 2.4 per cent of cases (or 1,200 people per 50,000, to use her measure). Not all of these would necessarily lead to bone marrow depletion, but it is cause for concern.

Concern that warrants more than two minutes per patient.

CARDURA (doxazosin)
Hypertension therapy
Cardura (doxazosin) had its fair share of side effects even before three doctors in England discovered another possible reaction that had never been recorded in any drugs reference work.

Cardura, manufactured by Pfizer, has been licensed for use in the UK and the US to treat hypertension (high blood pressure) and prostate problems.

Well-documented reactions include fatigue, headache and dizziness but, apart from some instances of anxiety and insomnia, few cases of psychiatric disorders have been reported.

But doctors at the Wirral Hospital on Merseyside reported in the British Medical Journal (BMJ, 1997; 314: 1869) a case of acute psychosis suffered by a 71-year-old woman while she was taking the drug.

She was admitted to the hospital's psychogeriatric ward after she began hearing noises which she claimed were coming from the walls of her house. Her psychosis started within a week or so of her doxazosin dosage being increased from 8 mg to 16 mg a day. The psychosis improved when the dose was adjusted back down to 8 mg.

The drug has also been the subject of one of America's largest ever class-action lawsuits. The action followed on from a study conducted by the National Heart Lung and Blood Institute that found that Cardura patients were twice as likely to be hospitalised for congestive heart failure and have a higher chance of suffering from other heart problems, such as stroke.

As a result, American heart specialists have been asked to think twice about prescribing Cardura for hypertension.

More common reactions to the drug include pain throughout the body, hypotension (low blood pressure), palpitations, abdominal pain, diarrhoea, oedema (fluid retention in tissues), sleepiness, respiratory disorder, urinary tract infection and increased sweating.

The doctors have reported the psychosis reaction to the Committee on Safety of Medicines although, currently, only 4 per cent of side effects from the drug are psychiatric symptoms.

CIPROXIN (ciprofloxacin hydrochloride)
Antibiotic for treating anthrax
Ciproxin is the marketing name in the UK for a drug that, for a while after the terrorist attacks on the World Trade Center, became the most wanted drug in the West.

Known in the US as Cipro, it is an antibiotic that has been approved in the

States as a treatment for inhaled anthrax. As such, during those uneasy days after the World Trade Center attacks, when several Americans died after having opened post contaminated with anthrax, virtually every doctor was being pressed for a prescription.

No wonder an NBC newscaster held up a bottle of pills and announced to the nation: "In Cipro we trust".

Unfortunately, his trust was misplaced. Cipro was rushed through the US drugs approval system 15 months earlier because of fears of a bioterrorist attack—and in so doing, the drug was never tested against anthrax in people. Its side effects can be alarming, and include dizziness, confusion, tremor, hallucinations, depression, an allergic reaction which can result in breathing difficulties, pain, inflammation or rupture of a tendon, and severe tissue inflammation of the colon.

None of this mattered in the rush to safeguard lives against terrorism but, within days, over one-fifth of the people in Florida who had been given Cipro were reporting side effects. Former patients were also telling newspapers how the drug had ruined their lives.

For the drug to be effective against anthrax, the patient has to take it for 60 days. This was unknown territory for a drug that had only been prescribed in the past for, at most, a 10-day regime. With hundreds of thousands of Americans suddenly embarking on the full 60-day procedure, the world's largest unregulated drugs trial has just been completed.

We await the results with interest.

CLARITYN (loratadine)

Hayfever remedy

Medicine is, of course, a holy alliance between doctor and patient, and the writing of the prescription is a little short of a sacrament.

So, imagine the horror of United Airlines passengers in the US who were offered a bag tag featuring an advert for Clarityn (loratadine), a prescription hayfever drug from Schering. They could also claim a $5 rebate certificate if they called a freefone (toll-free) number. The pitch is topped off with that immortal line from Irving Berlin: "Nothing but blue skies from now on".

What an airline is doing pushing a prescription drug nobody is quite sure. Perhaps it's the start of a new form of medical diagnosis, where airline staff can help the overstretched medical establishment. Passengers who overindulge in cream cakes while on board could be offered a cholesterol-lowering drug, while those in a long queue at check-in might be given a prescription for a stress-reducer.

But before any airline goes too far down this path, it might want to check the safety of the drug it's promoting. In one study of 300 children aged between six and 12 years, those given Clarityn syrup were more likely than the placebo group to suffer nervousness, wheezing, fatigue, abdominal pain, conjunctivitis, malaise and upper respiratory tract infections.

Other adverse reactions, reported in fewer than 2 per cent of patients, included flushing, back pain, eye pain, tinnitus, hypertension, hypotension, anorexia, constipation, toothache, vomiting, myalgia, insomnia and amnesia, and the list goes on. More seriously, perhaps, cases of hepatitis, jaundice and seizure have also been reported while people have been on the drug.

So, come fly the friendly skies of medicine . . .

CLOMID (clomiphene)
Infertility drug

Clomid (clomiphene) is a powerful and longstanding infertility drug but, of late, research has been suggesting that it can cause birth defects.

Those at risk are women who start taking the drug without realising they are already pregnant and women who become pregnant while taking the drug. The simple solution is for all women to have a pregnancy test before and during treatment with the drug. If she has already taken the drug, her pregnancy should be monitored carefully, reports medical journal Revue Prescrire (1999; 19: 40–1).

The manufacturer states that birth defects among users who are already pregnant are no more common than in the general population, although animal tests have suggested otherwise.

Fetal abnormalities that have been noted include, in order of frequency, heart lesions, Down's syndrome, clubfoot and gut lesions.

But a pregnancy check is not the only one that should be carried out before prescribing Clomid. Women who have ovarian cysts or abnormal vaginal bleeding should not be given the drug, nor should those with abnormal liver function.

One of the most common adverse reactions to the drug is visual disturbance, such as spots or flashes, and these increase in incidence the longer the drug is taken.

Another adverse reaction is ovarian hyperstimulation syndrome (OHSS), in which the ovaries become enlarged, or there may be gastrointestinal problems and, occasionally, hypotension.

Other reactions can include breast pain, headache and unusual uterine bleeding. Later trials have shown that it can also cause acne, migraine, heart problems and chest pain, liver problems, endometriosis and tinnitus.

The drug, however, is effective and can help pregnancy in 30 per cent of previously infertile women, but with the very real possibility of twins or triplets or, in a few cases, quintuplets!

CONDROTEC (naproxen/misoprostol)
NSAID for arthritis

Naproxen is an established NSAID (non-steroidal anti-inflammatory drug) for treating arthritis. But one of its main problems is that it can cause serious gastrointestinal problems, such as bleeding and ulcers.

Misoprostol is routinely given to naproxen patients who are most at risk from developing ulcers while taking an NSAID.

So the clever people at Searle have come up with a new antiarthritis drug called Condrotec, which mixes naproxen and misoprostol all in the same tablet. As the advert says: "Naproxen power with misoprostol protection."

But before the cigars are handed out, it's worth looking to see just how protective misoprostol can be. As regular readers will doubtless guess, the major reaction to misoprostol is . . . gastrointestinal problems. Although it will not cause ulcers, the drug can still bring on problems such as diarrhoea and abdominal pain. Women are particularly at risk as misoprostol can be responsible for a range of gynaecological complaints, such as spotting, cramps and other menstrual disorders.

Common reactions experienced by both sexes include nausea, flatulence, headache, dyspepsia, vomiting and constipation.

Turning to naproxen, the other reactions other than ulcers include serious kidney problems, liver abnormalities and fluid retention, the usual list of suspects linked to most every other NSAID.

Other common reactions include constipation, heartburn, headache, dizziness, vertigo, itching, tinnitus, visual disturbances, depression, insomnia, congestive heart failure and muscle pain.

Of course, there is the other vexed question of how the two drugs will interact with each other, especially as they are being taken at the same time. What little we do know is that misoprostol does not react with aspirin, but it is early days. Still, perhaps the manufacturer could throw something else into the cocktail if new reactions are discovered.

CORDARONE (amiodarone)
Powerful drug for irregular heartbeat (arrhythmia)

If you have a life-threatening condition, the chances are that the drug selected to treat you will be . . . life-threatening. Drastic measures for drastic times, you might say. Or perhaps: 'If the illness doesn't get you, the drugs will.'

Take, for instance, the drug Cordarone (amiodarone), perhaps more appropriately known in the UK as Cordarone X. It's one of a new generation of drugs for treating arrhythmias, or irregular heartbeat.

The *Physicians' Desk Reference* (*PDR*), the US drugs bible, warns that the drug has life-threatening side effects, and so is only suitable for patients with a life-threatening condition. The *PDR* recommends that the drug should be administered, initially at least, in hospital, and under very careful supervision. Only doctors who specialise in arrhythmia should prescribe the drug.

The warning was endorsed by a study that found that the drug also causes thyroid dysfunction. Among 92 patients, one-third developed thyroid side effects, which makes it particularly dangerous for people suffering with a congenital heart condition. Yes, that's right, the very people who are supposed to take the drug (Circulation, 1999; 100: 149–54).

The thyroid problem is a new one. Researchers also already knew that Cordarone produces fatal pulmonary toxicity in 10 per cent of all patients, while liver damage is common.

The manufacturer has also added to the warnings by announcing that the drug can affect the optic nerves, sometimes even leading to blindness.

Of course, like other similar drugs, it can make the arrhythmia worse, and has done so in around 5 per cent of patients. Significant heart block has been reported in a similar proportion of patients.

So, all in all, you could say the drug's not for the faint-hearted. But who then should take it?

COZAAR (losartan potassium)
Angiotensin blocker for hypertension
Cozaar (losartan potassium) is heralded by its manufacturer Merck Sharp & Dohme as being "the first of a new class" for treating hypertension, or high blood pressure.

The class in question is known as angiotensin-II receptor blockers, and is supposed to be a safer alternative to the ACE-inhibitor family. One test that bears out this theory found that losartan potassium did not trigger the dry cough usually associated with ACE inhibitors, which frequently gets so bad that treatment has to be stopped.

Around five million patients around the world have been treated with

Cozaar over three years, and with few side effects. Any effects, says the manufacturer, have been mild and transient, and most have had an incidence rate similar to a placebo; in other words, the effect could have happened, anyway.

So, has Merck produced the first perfect drug? Not if you're a pregnant woman still in your second or third trimester. Taking the drug could cause you to abort the baby, or it could be born with a serious handicap.

And, for the rest of the population, the argument that the drug's side effects are no worse than a placebo doesn't quite add up. Incidence of muscle cramping is much higher, as is dizziness, insomnia, sinusitis and upper respiratory infection.

The manufacturer also says the drug is well tolerated with others which, again, is not quite the case. Patients who are hypersensitive to aspirin and penicillin suffered swelling of the lips and eyelids, and facial rashes when given Cozaar.

Other reactions that have been observed include diarrhoea, muscle pain and migraine.

Despite this, Cozaar is probably a safer option than the ACE inhibitors, which may not be saying quite as much as the manufacturer would have you believe.

DESMOSPRAY (desmopressin)
Nasal spray to stop bedwetting
Desmopressin is the generic name of an antidiuretic hormone used as a nasal spray designed to stop bedwetting. It is marketed in the US by Rhone-Poulenc as DDAVP, and by Ferring as Desmospray in the UK.

It can be taken by children as young as six years of age, who are advised to take 10 mcg (microgrammes) in each nostril before going to sleep. The ideal dosage is arrived at only by trial and error, with the minimum dosage being 10 mcg, going up to 40 mcg. The dose sometimes has to be increased after six months' usage, when the effects seem to diminish. Any patient who has taken the drug that long has gone further than medicine; trials have tested the drug and reactions for only four to eight weeks of use.

A dose that is too high can result in headaches, nausea, nasal congestion, rhinitis, flushing, abdominal cramps, nosebleeds, sore throat, cough and upper respiratory infection.

Because it is an antidiuretic, desmopressin has the effect of reducing urine output as well as the movement of blood plasma. This latter effect can, on rare occasions, result in seizures and even coma.

Another major worry, particularly among smaller children, is water intoxication, which can occur if a child drinks too much water before going to bed while on the drug.

More common reactions include depression, dizziness, rash, conjunctivitis and other eye disorders.

People who should not be given the drug include those with a history of coronary problems, and those with fluid imbalance, such as cystic fibrosis sufferers. Trials on pregnant women and breastfeeding mothers have never been carried out.

The drug can also be supplied intravenously, although cases of anaphylactic (allergic) shock have been reported.

DEXEDRINE (dextroamphetamine)
Amphetamine for weight loss and ADHD
Parents who wonder just what illicit use of drugs can do to their children need only cast an eye across the adverse reactions with Dexedrine to get the picture.

Dexedrine is an amphetamine, designed by SmithKline Beecham to help people lose weight, but is often abused by young people as one of the 'speed' drugs.

Of course, young people can claim to have ADHD or hyperactivity, and they'll get a prescription in a shot. Like Ritalin, another amphetamine, it's being heralded as a successful therapy to treat America's—and, more recently, Britain's—young.

A patient on Dexedrine will eventually develop a tolerance to the drug, at which point treatment should be stopped. Dosage, which ranges from 5 to 60 mg a day in divided doses, should not be increased.

It should never be given to people with a history of glaucoma, high blood pressure, heart disease or overactive thyroid.

Because the drug contains tartrazine, it may trigger asthma or some other bronchial reaction.

Other reactions include palpitations, raised blood pressure, raised heart rate and cardiomyopathy, or heart disease, although this occurs only when the dose is exceeded. The central nervous system can also be affected, and symptoms then include overstimulation, restlessness, insomnia, nervous tics and tremors. Diarrhoea and constipation can also occur.

Overdosage depends on the individual's own metabolism, but reactions can occur with as little as 2 mg although, normally, 30 mg would have to be taken before severe reactions are noted. Reactions at these dosages have included hallucinations, panic attacks and nausea. A fatal dose is usually preceded by convulsions and coma.

DIDRONEL (etidronate)
Drug for osteoporosis of the spine

Didronel PMO, a combination of the drug etidronate and calcium, is licensed specifically for the treatment of established vertebral osteoporosis, or serious bone-thinning of the spine.

The manufacturer Norwich Eaton was so enthusiastic about the benefits of the drug that it ran a campaign that appeared to urge doctors to prescribe it for wrist and hip fractures, and to prevent osteoporosis in women after the menopause, despite the fact that the drug is not licensed for such use. The Consumers' Association responded angrily to such apparent poetic licence being taken, claiming that the product was being "illegally promoted".

When taken continuously, studies show that etidronate can cause osteomalacia, an adult form of rickets caused by lack of vitamin D. In 1976, researchers found that etidronate at a dose of 20 mg per kilogram of body weight every day for six to 12 months did, indeed, reduce thinning of the bones. But it also caused a reduction in bone mineralisation (Clin Pharmacol Ther, 1976; 20: 593–604). Didronel PMO is designed to be taken intermittently in conjunction with calcium carbonate, supposedly to prevent osteomalacia. However, at least one study suggests that, when taken in this way, etidronate fails to prevent the loss of vertebral bone (Miner Electrolyte Metabol, 1988; 66: 747–53).

Even if the drug does work, you may just be substituting one bone problem for another. An editorial in The Lancet (5 May 1990) warns that the length of time the drug stays in the body "could theoretically lead to increased amounts of 'old bone' in the very long term because of reduced remodelling". Etidronate's established side effects include angioedema (fluid retention of the blood vessels), nausea, diarrhoea, abdominal pain, constipation and vomiting. There have also been reports of patients developing white blood cell abnormalities.

DIFLUCAN (fluconazole)
Therapy for yeast problems

Diflucan (fluconazole) was sold to doctors as the 'elegant' way to deal with vaginal thrush (yeast infection). A single 150-mg pill would rid their patients of this common annoyance without the messiness, leakage and vaginal irritation of the usual creams and gels.

This assurance of safety has caused many doctors to use Diflucan for early treatment of systemic *Candida* infection, particularly patients who are immunosuppressed or receiving chemotherapy drugs. Because they can be given orally as systemic drugs (unlike nystatin and amphotericin B, which are highly toxic if they pass through your liver rather than simply your gut), fluconazole (and the other 'azoles' ketoconazole and itraconazole) are now the drugs of choice for systemic *Candida* infections.

However, some studies have shown that urinary tract and *Candida* infections can develop resistance to fluconazole, particularly in those receiving oral steroids (Lancet, 30 March, 19 January, 29 June 1991), or cause other *Candida* species, such as *Candida krusei*, to overgrow (N Engl J Med, 31 October 1991).

As for side effects, studies have shown that fluconazole can cause rash, the sometimes fatal skin disorder Stevens–Johnson syndrome, nausea and vomiting, headache, seizures and, rarely, hepatitis. Because of the potential for Stevens–Johnson syndrome, even in patients given a short course of 150 mg a day, doctors at Bronovo Hospital in the Hague, Netherlands, cautioned: "We believe that fluconazole should be used with caution for conditions that can also be treated with topical non-absorbable antifungal drugs" (Lancet, 13 July 1991).

It is also known to interact with drugs for hypoglycaemia, steroids, carbamazepine, phenobarbital, the thiazide diuretics and cyclosporin.

DUTONIN (nefazodone)
New family of antidepressant

Dutonin, an antidepressant, was launched with the claim that it is as effective as Prozac, but with far fewer side effects. But the marketing men may have to do a rethink following new reports from the US that the drug could cause liver failure so severe as to result in a transplant or death.

The US drugs regulator, the Food and Drug Administration, knows that the problem affects about 1 in 60,000 patients but, because of serious underreporting, recognises that the problem is much worse.

Patients with liver disease shouldn't take the drug, and doctors in the US have been put on the alert for warning signs such as jaundice, anorexia and gastrointestinal complaints.

Dutonin (nefazodone), called Serzone in North America, was heralded as a new kind of antidepressant when the FDA licensed it in 1994. Unlike SSRIs like Prozac that boost serotonin levels, and tricyclics that block serotonin receptors, Dutonin is supposed to do both, as well as block the receptors called 5-HT$_2$, which are among those most likely to cause depression.

Despite the early claims of fewer side effects than Prozac, 16 per cent of patients in a trial of 3,496 patients had to discontinue treatment because of an adverse reaction. The most common reactions included nausea, dizziness, insomnia, asthenia (feeling weak) and agitation.

Other common side effects have included sleepiness, dry mouth, constipation, blurred and abnormal vision, lightheadedness and confusion.

It can also be dangerous to take Dutonin with other drugs, especially antihistamines like Seldane and Hismanal, as the combination can increase blood drug levels to the point of being life-threatening.

When Dutonin was launched, doctors were not convinced that it was as effective as the SSRIs. They now have a further reason to pause before writing the prescription.

EFEXOR (venlafaxine hydrochloride)
Antidepressant

Of late, the marketing men at several drug companies have been mounting an assault on Prozac, the antidepressant that seems to have become a lifeline for a nervous generation.

As Prozac is seen as a powerful agent that can seemingly alter personalities, the approach of its rivals is surprising. In so many words, they're saying that their antidepressant is more powerful, and faster-acting, than Prozac. Prozac is for sissies, perhaps?

Take, for example, the claims for Efexor (which inexplicably develops a second 'f' for the US market). It is "nearly twice as effective as fluoxetine [Prozac] in eradicating the symptoms of depression", an advertisement to doctors states, quoting a scientific poster presented at a conference in Vienna. A poster? Stranger and stranger.

Posters aside, the effectiveness of Efexor (venlafaxine hydrochloride) for long-term use of more than six weeks has not been proved (*Physicians' Desk Reference*, 1998).

But what is not in doubt is that, as a powerful antidepressant, it comes with a raft of side effects. The major worry is over patients who have been taking monoamine oxidase inhibitors (MAOIs) and who then immediately start a course of Efexor. Serious adverse reactions in these people have been reported, including tremor, nausea, vomiting, flushing, dizziness, seizures and death.

Even without previous MAOI usage, 19 per cent of Efexor patients had to stop treatment prematurely because of some adverse reaction. The most common problem was nausea, but others included insomnia, dizziness, nervousness, dry mouth, anxiety and sweating.

Like Prozac, abnormal personality changes have also been noted. In one trial, 11 per cent of patients developed anorexia, and significant weight loss was also reported in those who did not intend it. A 5 per cent loss in body weight was reported in 6 per cent of patients.

ELTROXIN (levothyroxine sodium)
Thyroid treatment

The different approaches of the UK and US drugs regulators have been noted more than once by us. A current case in point concerns the thyroid replacement drugs and, in particular, levothyroxine sodium, marketed in the UK as Eltroxin and, in the US, as Synthroid.

In the US, the Food and Drug Administration (FDA) is seriously considering a withdrawal of the drug because it has "a history of problems" and cannot be recognised as "safe and effective". The drug is also the subject of a raft of class-action lawsuits in the US.

Despite this, the Committee on Safety of Medicines, the UK drugs watchdog, appears to have no such qualms.

The drug treats hypothyroidism, when the thyroid underperforms, by drip-feeding exact amounts of synthetic thyroxine, a major hormone produced by the thyroid. It's a delicate balance and one that often goes askew and, when it does, the thyroid will either not do all it should or go into overdrive. The FDA noted that: "Synthroid has not been reliably potent and stable." As a result, "patients receive tablets that are filled with a product of unpredictable potency" and so "therapy with thyroxine sodium is neither safe nor effective."

Most of the side effects of Synthroid and Eltroxin are related to overdosage, which causes symptoms of hyperthyroidism (an overactive thyroid). These include heart pain, irregular heart rhythm, palpitations, muscle cramping, tremors, restlessness, excitability, insomnia, headache, sweating, excessive weight loss and muscular weakness.

In its 40 years of use in the US, Synthroid has been the subject of numerous product recalls because of dosage problems. Even so, it is the third most prescribed drug in America—yet the FDA is prepared to withdraw it if necessary.

We hope that the Committee on Safety of Medicines is watching.

EMBLON (tamoxifen)
Breast cancer therapy
The breast cancer drug tamoxifen—marketed in the UK as Emblon, Noltam and Tamofen, and as Nolvadex in the US and the UK—has been enjoying some favourable press comment.

Tamoxifen, prescribed for over 20 years, is a hormone drug designed to slow the spread of cancer by blocking oestrogen production.

Now, a number of newspapers have been hailing it as a miracle. This sudden support has been sparked by fears in the UK that a major study of the drug among 15,000 healthy women may be jeopardised by the suspension of a similar trial in the US.

The US trial was stopped following allegations that the trial leader, Dr Bernard Fisher, had failed to explain, in the consent form that trial members signed, all the dangers of the drug as highlighted in previous research.

These trials, along with similar studies in 14 other countries, have been testing tamoxifen as a cancer preventative among healthy women. While the general consensus is that tamoxifen's benefits outweigh the risks among women already with breast cancer, there is a growing list of side effects that justifiably cause concern, particularly if given to a woman with no symptoms.

Six American women have died from endometrial (womb lining) cancer after taking the drug, which tallies with a recent Dutch study that concluded that women taking tamoxifen more than doubled their risk of developing the cancer (Lancet, 19 February 1994). An earlier, major Swedish study had put the risk at greater than six times (Lancet, 1989; *i*: 117–20).

Other concerns include the dangers of liver cancer. In tests with rats, 11.5 per cent developed the cancer at normal doses, and this increased to 71 per cent at higher doses (J Nat Cancer Inst, 1991; 83: 1450–9).

Other side effects, listed in the US *Physicians' Desk Reference*, include eye problems such as corneal changes and cataracts, the production of excessive calcium, vaginal bleeding, hot flashes, nausea (reported in a quarter of all cases) and skin rash.

EPILIM (sodium valproate)
Epilepsy treatment
Sodium valproate, also known as valproic acid and marketed under the brand names Epilim, or Depakene or Depakote in the US, is a drug used in the treatment of epilepsy. It is also being discussed as a possible treatment of autism (Ann Intern Med, 1 February 1994).

It is a powerful drug that brings with it a host of possible side effects, the most dangerous of which is its capacity to cause potentially fatal liver failure in some patients. However, the strength of the warning of this danger will depend on which side of the Atlantic you happen to live, with Britain far more lax about disclosure of side effects than the US.

In the US, prescribing doctors are forcibly reminded of this potential by the *Physicians' Desk Reference*. In the *PDR*, the entry for the drug opens with the words: "WARNING: HEPATIC FAILURE RESULTING IN FATALITIES HAS OCCURRED IN PATIENTS RECEIVING VALPROIC ACID."

However, the UK's equivalent of the *PDR*, *The Medicines Compendium* (previously *The Data Sheet Compendium*), is far more circumspect. Its reference to potentially fatal liver damage is tucked away midway through the text.

The *PDR* is unequivocal in its attitude towards giving valproate to children under two years of age who have associated problems, saying baldly: "IN THIS PATIENT GROUP, IT SHOULD BE USED WITH EXTREME CAUTION AND AS A SOLE AGENT. THE BENEFITS OF SEIZURE CONTROL SHOULD BE WEIGHED AGAINST THE RISKS". The *TMC* says only: "Monotherapy [treatment with only one type of drug] is to be preferred."

The *PDR* continues on in capital letters about the potential of valproate to cause spina bifida in babies born to mothers taking the drug, and severe central nervous system depression if given with barbiturates. It also warns of the possibility of breakthrough seizures if used in combination with phenytoin. The *TMC*, on the other hand, makes no mention of the latter two risks.

Both directories agree that all patients taking this drug should have their liver function monitored before and during treatment. They warn that doctors should not rely simply on the results of laboratory tests (which may not always show up as abnormal), but take a detailed medical history of the patient and conduct a thorough physical examination.

EVISTA (raloxifene)
Non-hormonal treatment for the menopause
The clever marketing people in the drugs industry managed to convince everyone that the menopause is a disease. Having done that, they were then able to offer a 'cure', initially in the shape of hormone replacement therapy (HRT).

Then some troublemakers started having doubts, saying that it could cause breast cancer. So what happened? Women started questioning their GPs, and wanted a more natural 'cure'.

As every woman will pass through the menopause, it's not a market you want to give up without a fight.

One of the first to show its hand was Eli Lilly, which has developed raloxifene (marketed in the UK as Evista). Yes, they say, menopause is still a disease and, yes, HRT may indeed be a problem. So how about a non-hormonal treatment that will protect you against osteoporosis while not stimulating breast and endometrial tissues?

One of the first major studies into the drug, tested on 601 postmenopausal women, gave it a glowing reference. Daily therapy could increase bone mineral density and lower blood concentrations of cholesterol, without stimulating the endometrium.

They also mentioned, in passing, that 25 per cent of the women dropped out of the study (N Engl J Med, 1997; 337: 1641–7). Incidents of breast pain and hot flashes in particular were noted, but they were no worse than those experienced in the group being given a placebo.

Eli Lilly has discovered in separate trials that raloxifene can cause thrombosis, pulmonary embolism, leg cramps and hot flushes, so perhaps these were the other reasons why the women stopped taking the drug.

At least there was no mention of breast cancer.

FELDENE (piroxicam)
NSAID for arthritis

Feldene (generic name: piroxicam) seems to be one of those drugs that people either hate or really loathe. Manufactured by Pfizer, it's a non-steroidal anti-inflammatory drug (NSAID) designed to treat both osteoarthritis and rheumatoid arthritis.

It's rarely been out of the news. Most recently, it caught the attention of the US Food and Drug Administration (FDA) because Pfizer had failed to report cases of adverse drug reactions to the drug within the statutory 15 days. Pfizer's reports were between 70 and 500 days late.

The Health Research Group, the American medical watchdog group, petitioned the FDA to have Feldene banned for the over-60s. The Group claims the drug has caused serious side effects, and "numerous deaths", especially in older people. People over the age of 60 are more likely than others to suffer stomach and intestinal bleeding, ulcers and perforations, the Group reports.

The Canadian drug regulators, worried about adverse reactions to Feldene, have halved the recommended dose to just 10 mg a day, whereas the British and American authorities have stuck to the 20-mg dosage.

Extensive trials revealed that 30 per cent of users on 20 mg a day suffer some side effect. Gastrointestinal symptoms, such as bleeding, ulcers and perforation, occurred in 20 per cent of users, while others reported dizziness, headaches, vertigo, tinnitus, depression, insomnia, swollen eyes, hair loss, jaundice and rashes.

In all, the American *Physicians' Desk Reference* (*PDR*) lists around 110 possible side effects. In a note to patients, the *PDR* states: "Feldene, like other drugs of its class, is not free of side effects", a sentence presumably up for the Jack Benny Pithy Understatement Award. To doctors, it advises counselling to patients of the potential risks.

FOSAMAX (alendronate sodium)
Treatment for postmenopausal osteoporosis

Osteoporosis is a common problem among postmenopausal women. It is a disease that results in progressive bone loss, and the risk of hip fracture for women aged between 50 and 90 increases 50-fold, while the risk of spinal fracture increases by 15 to 30 times.

Both diet and moderate exercise have been scientifically proven to be very effective in combating osteoporosis.

Those who would rather not take direct control of their own health might prefer to try the drug Fosamax (alendronate sodium). Alendronate binds to the bone while restricting the effects of osteoporosis, although it does slow the growth of new bone. This means your body doesn't have the bone turnover that it would before the menopause.

The manufacturer, Merck, has recently been trumpeting the virtues of Fosamax following the results of the FIT (Fracture Intervention Trial), which involved 2,027 postmenopausal women (Lancet, 1996; 348: 1535–41). The trial showed that the drug reduced hip fractures by 51 per cent and new vertebral (spinal) fractures by 47 per cent. Equally impressive, it has similar adverse reactions to placebo.

A trial in the US of 1,800 postmenopausal women came to similar conclusions about its safety. However, 4.1 per cent of patients had to stop treatment because of adverse reactions, which included abdominal pain, nausea, dyspepsia and musculoskeletal pain. Women with kidney problems have been warned not to take the drug, mainly because the body will not be so efficient in processing it so that too much of it may stay in the system.

Merck recommends that patients should also maintain an "adequate" calcium diet. They might also have suggested a good exercise regimen as well perhaps, then their patients may not even need the drug.

GENTICIN (gentamicin)
Antibiotic for infections
Don't just read the label—watch the patient, too. Enough vigilant doctors and healthcare professionals in the US reported unexpected reactions among patients to gentamicin, a broad-spectrum antibiotic used to treat serious infections, that the drug regulator, the Food and Drug Administration (FDA), started to investigate.

Patients complained of fever within hours of receiving the intravenous (iv) version of the drug, a symptom that had not been widely reported before and so was not among the likely reactions listed by the manufacturer.

In all, 155 patients reported a range of reactions, including chills, shaking or shivering, rigours, fever, a sudden rapid heartbeat, hypertension and hypotension, and respiratory problems.

Twelve of the 155 suffered reactions so serious that they were treated in hospital, and five needed intensive care.

The worry for the FDA was that all these cases occurred with the once-daily iv version—now used by most hospitals for convenience—which had never been tested by its scientific review and so was not included in the standard product labelling.

Initially, FDA investigators thought the once-daily dose was too high (the usual dosage is smaller amounts three times a day), but discovered that several bulk supplies of the drug contained high levels of an endotoxin (toxins derived from the outer membranes of certain bacteria).

The supplies came from the same manufacturer, and the FDA issued an immediate ban on importing products from the firm. New supplies from a different manufacturer have been reintroduced without incident (N Engl J Med, 2000; 342: 1658–9).

But even without manufacturing faults, gentamicin comes with its own problems. It can seriously damage the kidneys as well as the nervous system (reactions to look out for include numbness, skin-tingling, muscle-twitching and convulsions).

IMIGRAN (sumatriptan)
Migraine treatment
Sumatriptan is the latest wonder drug for treating the misery of migraine

headache. It was launched by Glaxo under the brand name of Imigran.

As with most wonder drugs, sumatriptan is hugely expensive: £8 for one tablet, or £20 for one injection. Despite the cost, studies show that sumatriptan tablets don't work in up to one-third of patients, and up to one-sixth of those receiving the injection derive no benefit. Where an initial injection hasn't worked, there is no evidence that a second shot will make any difference.

Similarly, with tablet sumatriptan, studies suggest that a 100-mg dose is the optimal amount, and that larger doses don't afford greater relief. Even with those helped by the drug, an alarmingly high proportion—higher than that seen with other antimigraine drugs—suffer repeat attacks.

A Swedish migraine clinic reports that 53 per cent of patients "have had recurrences within five to 10 hours after almost every treated attack" (Lancet, 10 October 1992).

The same Swedish clinic reported that 70 per cent of those injected with sumatriptan suffered some side effects, most commonly neck pain or stiffness, tiredness, tightness or pressure across the chest, injection site reactions and tingling. The same range of side effects was reported in controlled trials of 4,859 patients.

These controlled trials also showed that oral (tablet) sumatriptan causes vomiting, taste disturbances, malaise, fatigue, dizziness and vertigo, drowsiness and chest symptoms.

Out of that catalogue of side effects, it is the chest symptoms that are causing the most concern. Sumatriptan causes blood vessels in the brain to constrict and so theoretically helps stave off a migraine attack.

But there is growing concern that the drug has a similar constricting effect on circulation around the heart. The British Medical Journal (19 September 1992) reports two cases of serious abnormal heartbeat linked with sumatriptan. In one case, a 42-year-old woman with no history of heart disease collapsed when her heart stopped within three minutes of being injected with the drug.

Not surprisingly, the UK Committee on Safety of Medicines warns against the use of this drug in patients with coronary artery disease.

It should also be avoided by those with angina and high blood pressure, and "used cautiously" in patients with conditions that predispose them towards heart disease (Drug Ther Bull, 26 October 1992). Children, elderly people, pregnant and lactating women should not take sumatriptan.

Our verdict: darkened rooms and ice packs preferred.

IMURAN (azathioprine)

Immunosuppressant

Azathioprine, like cyclosporin, is an immunosuppressant drug originally designed to stop rejection in organ transplant patients. It tinkers with the body's immune function, leaving it susceptible to all manner of infections.

Azathioprine is an extremely powerful and dangerous drug. We are amazed that any doctor should suggest administering it to a child as young as two, as we discovered in one case. It is particularly alarming that it should be recommended as a treatment for ulcerative colitis, given that its side effects include gastrointestinal problems, such as severe nausea, vomiting and anorexia. According to the US *Physicians' Desk Reference*, these symptoms may be accompanied by diarrhoea, rash, fever, malaise, muscle pain, elevations in liver enzymes and, occasionally, raised blood pressure. It also causes duodenal ulcers and intestinal haemorrhage.

Its potential for harm is so great that the *PDR* says in a special black-box warning that chronic immunosuppression leads to an increased risk of tumours, particularly those of the lymphatic system. Doctors prescribing this drug should be very familiar with this potential, it says.

Another toxic effect is suppression of bone marrow function, which can lead to a reduced white blood cell count and anaemia. The *PDR* recommends that patients be given complete blood counts, including platelets, every week during the first month of treatment.

Azathioprine has been shown to disturb kidney and liver function. It has also been shown to cause birth defects affecting the skeleton and internal organs in animals, and chromosome damage in humans.

Patients given the drug after transplants also have an increased incidence of skin cancer, particularly on skin exposed to the sun. "Patients should be cautioned against undue sun exposure and skin should be examined at regular intervals," says *The Medicines Compendium*.

It adds that there have also been rare cases of lung disease and meningitis.

LAMICTAL (lamotrigine)

Epileptic drug

The antiepileptic drug lamotrigine (marketed as Lamictal) is yet another drug being used for a different purpose than was originally intended.

Danish researchers have found that it relieves severe pain following a stroke. They tested it on 30 patients and found that 200 mg per day reduced pain scores by around 30 per cent.

The only other drug with a proven effect on central poststroke pain

(CPSP) is amitriptyline, which comes with a range of serious side effects, point out researchers.

Not unlike lamotrigine, in fact. The drug is honoured with a black-box warning in the American drug bible, the *Physicians' Desk Reference*. The warning states that up to one in every 1,000 lamotrigine adult patients could develop a life-threatening rash, an incidence rate that is greatly increased among children. "Although benign rashes also occur with Lamictal, it is not possible to predict reliably which rashes will prove to be life-threatening," warns the *PDR*.

A significant point, and one apparently overlooked by research team head Troels Jensen, who said: "Patients tolerated lamotrigine well in our study; the only side effect is a rash . . ." (Neurology, 2001; 56: 184–90).

Death aside, other effects of lamotrigine include dizziness, headache, blurred vision, nausea and vomiting. Less common reactions have included multiorgan failure, sudden and unexplained death, and blindness.

"Lamotrigine is clearly not a wonder drug," says Willem Meijler at the Comprehensive Cancer Centre in Groningen, the Netherlands, and clearly a master of the understatement, "but in this group of patients [in the Danish study], it's a major step."

The last word is reserved for Troels Jensen. "Lamotrigine is a welcome addition in our arsenal," he says.

Let's hope that is not a rash statement.

LAMISIL (terbinafine)
Antifungal drug
Terbinafine (Lamisil) is given orally to treat fungal skin and nail infections. Well-documented side effects include stomach problems, nausea, loss of appetite, abdominal pain, diarrhoea, skin eruptions and kidney dysfunction, including jaundice.

It can also cause joint and muscle pain and, as it is excreted in breast milk, should never be taken by breastfeeding mothers.

But perhaps the most serious reactions, which have warranted a public health alert from the American drugs regulator, the Food and Drug Administration, is a link to congestive heart failure and hepatic reactions. An estimated 11 people have died from liver complications while taking the drug, and two others have needed liver transplants. The FDA's concerns about liver complications do not extend to the cream and solution formulations of the drug.

Doctors in Canada also reported a previously unrecorded side effect linked to the drug, which led to two previously healthy individuals being hospitalised (Med Monitor, 17 September 1997). Three patients with stable psoriasis, where the skin erupts in red, scaly lesions, found their skin condition became much worse. In one case, a patient whose rash was previously confined to her hands, feet and nails found that it had spread to her trunk and arms.

In another, within three weeks of taking the drug for a nail infection, a woman was covered in pustular psoriasis and needed hospital treatment.

In a fourth case, after taking terbinafine, a patient with no personal or family history of the condition also ended up in hospital with pustular psoriasis.

Doctors should be more careful about dishing out this drug, concludes the Medical Monitor. Malformed nails "can be due to fungal infections or psoriasis or even both, which cannot be clinically distinguished". A diagnosis should be confirmed before antifungal treatment is started. "There is no point in risking side effects when the dystrophy is due to psoriasis rather than infection," it concludes.

It's also been at the centre of a major dispensing error in US pharmacies. Patients have been given Lamictal, the antiepileptic drug, instead of Lamisil. The confusion has been caused because of the closeness of the two names. As a result, patients have been suffering serious adverse reactions—and, of course, not getting the treatment they've been prescribed.

LARIAM (mefloquine hydrochloride)
Malaria drug
Lariam (mefloquine hydrochloride), the antimalarial drug produced by Hoffman-La Roche, has rarely been out of the news since its introduction in the 1980s.

The flames of controversy were fanned once again with the first reported death from the drug. A six-year-old girl died in an English hospital after returning from a holiday in Nigeria. She suffered a severe reaction, known as toxic epidermal necrolysis, and died after 19 days in hospital from a heart attack.

This follows on from a class-action lawsuit against the Swiss manufacturer by 300 Britons, who are all claiming severe and long-term effects after taking the drug. They are still suffering hallucinations, anxiety attacks, seizures and severe mood swings, they say.

Many travellers are refusing to take the drug, and British Airways has issued a warning to all staff about Lariam.

Lariam is considered to be the most powerful of all the antimalarials, and is designed as a preventative against, and as treatment for, resistant strains of malaria caught in sub-Sahara Africa, such as *Plasmodium falciparum* and *P. vivax*.

Because it is taken just once a week, Lariam tends to stay in the system for a long time. This means there can be a rapid buildup, and adverse reactions are experienced quite early on.

Patient groups in America have reported a litany of adverse reactions that have lasted for several years.

Hoffman-La Roche says that the effects of the drug on patients suffering from malaria are indistinguishable from the disease itself. As a preventative (prophylaxis), reactions can include vomiting, dizziness, nausea, fever, headache, chills, skin rash, tinnitus, hair loss, emotional problems and seizures. One patient suffered a heart attack after taking just one tablet.

To that long list must now be added another: death.

L-DOPA (dopamine)
Parkinson's disease treatment

Levodopa, or L-dopa, is the cornerstone of conventional treatment for Parkinson's disease, particularly among the over-70s. Other drugs are usually tried first on younger sufferers because of the serious side effects that can be triggered by the drug

Early side effects include nausea or vomiting, although practitioners say these pass fairly quickly as the body builds up tolerance to the drug. Others include hypotension (sudden lowering of blood pressure), aggravation of peptic ulcers, sweating attacks, and discoloration of urine and sweat.

The more serious reactions (as if those were not serious enough) include impairment of motor skills, heart irregularities, and mental changes, including paranoia sometimes leading to suicide. Convulsions have also occurred, albeit rarely.

The side effects admitted by the manufacturer in reference works such as the *Physicians' Desk Reference* (1995) read more like a litany of common and not-so-common complaints, too numerous to list here. A partial list includes nightmares, insomnia, headache, numbness, fatigue, euphoria, muscle twitching, diarrhoea, constipation, skin rash, blurred vision and weight gain or loss.

The biggest problem is trying to sort out the appropriate individual dose of the drug. Too little and the patient freezes, statue like; too much and the patient goes wild with uncontrollable movement.

And within 5–10 years, the drug stops working as patients lose their ability to convert L-dopa.

LIPOSTAT (pravastatin sodium)
Statin to lower cholesterol

Pravastatin sodium (Lipostat in the UK, Pravachol in the US), one of a new breed of 'statin' cholesterol-lowering drugs, is using a different marketing ploy to increase the drug's market share—flattery.

A new advertising campaign follows the line that pravastatin is the clear choice for someone with a logical, scientific mind—in other words, your family doctor.

The drug was given an enormous boost by the findings of the West of Scotland Coronary Prevention Study (WOSCOPS) of 6,595 men, who had never suffered a heart attack, given the drug, a change of diet or a placebo.

The drug was found to reduce the rate of a first heart attack by 31 per cent, compared with the other two groups and, as the trial was the 'gold standard' double-blind, placebo-controlled variety, it was a result to satisfy the most scientific of minds (Circulation, 1995; 92: 2419–25).

So successful was the trial, in fact, that over half of all patients now on the drug are women. A few, probably completely unscientific, commentators pointed out that any success recorded in men could not automatically be transferred to women.

And others, probably with hopelessly illogical minds, found that the group in the trial who were not given the drug seemed to suffer a far higher incidence of heart attack than average. So were these people less healthy than average, thus unfairly boosting the beneficial effects of the drug? A foolish question, of course, no doubt framed by someone far better at woodwork than science at school.

Then there are the adverse reactions that the drug can cause, such as heart pain, skin rashes, heartburn and fatigue, and the logic of choosing pravastatin becomes overwhelming, if not scientific.

LIVIAL (tibolone)
HRT

Livial (tibolone) is "the only HRT licensed to improve mood and libido", purrs the copyline of the ad aimed at your GP. The James Bond analogy is coupled with a very happy couple, smiling contendedly in bed. We know what they've been doing, presumably thanks to Livial, although they both look far too young to be worried about their menopausal years.

Perhaps they've just been on the phone to her mother, who has told them how Livial has changed her life. And perhaps their smiles are not so much from happiness, but from a wry concern. "She thinks she's licensed to improve her mood and libido, but has she any idea what the adverse reactions are with this drug?" they could be saying to each other.

And mother should be worried. Livial has been reported to cause a change in body weight and to trigger dizzy spells, rashes, itching, increased facial hair (good for disguises if you are a James Bond type, we suppose), headaches, migraine and visual disturbances, stomach upsets and abdominal pain, depression, oedema and musculoskeletal pain.

Livial, which is entirely synthetic (made from petrol-refinery sources), most definitely does not cause cancer, as do the more conventional HRTs, says the manufacturer but, then again, since studies are ongoing, nobody can yet be sure.

Like most HRTs, it should be carefully monitored by your GP. If bleeding starts and continues for a long time, your doctor should investigate. One worry is that it might start a thromboembolism, a concern shared with most HRT drugs, or cause liver malfunction, possibly leading to jaundice.

So, although mother may be beside herself because she is licensed to . . ., she needs to know that it always comes with a risk.

Just ask James Bond. He knows we don't really get to live twice.

LOSEC (ompeprazole)
Anti-ulcer treatment

Omeprazole—marketed as Losec in the UK—is touted as an improvement on older-style antiulcer drugs. Its manufacturer, the drug company Merck, is so certain of its benefits that it has been running a series of ads in the medical press knocking a rival ulcer treatment, Zantac (ranitidine), manufactured by another drug giant, Glaxo. "IF YOUR ZANTAC PATIENTS AREN'T COMPLETELY SYMPTOM-FREE AFTER WEEK 4, TURN TO PAGE XX". On turning to the appropriate page, doctors will find a two-page ad for Losec, insisting that this is the drug that succeeds where others have failed.

Losec is a new-style drug—a proton pump inhibitor—which stops the production of stomach acid to give the ulcer a chance to heal.

No doubt the campaign's message will filter down through doctors to patients. What may not reach such a wide audience, however, is the manufacturer's warning accompanying the ad that this drug has been shown to produce cancer in animals. "In long-term (two-year) studies in rats, omeprazole produced a dose-related increase in gastric carcinoid tumours," runs the warning. It adds that more research is needed to "rule out the possibility of an increased risk for the development of tumours in humans receiving long-term therapy with Losec."

That may be one reason why Losec is recommended only for short-term usage. "The efficacy of Losec used for longer than 8 weeks . . . has not been established," says the manufacturer.

Problems identified in US clinical trials include chest pain, raised blood pressure, liver failure (rarely), and psychic disturbances like hallucinations and insomnia. A 77-year-old man developed "painful nocturnal erections" lasting up to 36 hours while being treated with the drug (Lancet, 19 October 1991).

LOTRONEX (alosetron hydrochloride)
IBS treatment

GlaxoWellcome's drug Lotronex (alosetron hydrochloride) for irritable bowel syndrome (IBS) was withdrawn from the US market after just nine months, following reports of five deaths among patients. In all, the Food and Drug Administration, the US's drug regulator, received 70 reports of serious adverse reactions.

Yet, in an extraordinary *volte face*, the FDA advisory panel recommended that the drug be reintroduced, but with restrictions on who could prescribe it and provided that patients are carefully followed (Lancet, 2002; 359: 1491).

Their recommendation, which may not be endorsed by the FDA, was welcomed by Glaxo as "a very positive step forward for patients who need this drug."

Its withdrawal was all the more remarkable as Lotronex was chosen as the first drug to come with a full treatment guide under 'patient power' regulation. The guide warned that the principal side effect discovered in trials was constipation.

Hailed as "a promising aid for irritable bowel syndrome" (Drug Infoline, December 1999), a 12-week trial of 370 IBS sufferers found that the drug was effective among women compared with a placebo.

As well as being a drug intended only for women, it was also only supposed to treat the diarrhoea form of IBS.

Strangely, the trial did not pick up the serious adverse reactions that were soon being reported to the FDA. These reports centred around cases of intestinal damage resulting from reduced blood flow to the intestine, and severely obstructed or ruptured bowels, a complication of severe constipation.

Within four months of its release, six women needed hospital treatment and three of those underwent surgery, after being on the drug.

By the time GlaxoWellcome agreed to withdraw the drug, 34 patients had been treated in hospital, 10 others had undergone surgery and three had died. Two other deaths were not conclusively linked to the drug.

Dr Sidney Wolfe, of the consumer watchdog group Public Citizen, said that in clinical trials, there had been little difference in effectiveness between Lotronex and placebo. He was concerned that the FDA advisory panel's recommendation would lead to more patient deaths.

More worrying, why did the clinical trials not discover the possibly fatal reactions, and to what benefit, therefore, are 'patient power' leaflets?

LUSTRAL (sertraline)
Powerful antidepressant

"Reason to be cheerful" chirrups the advertisement for sertraline, a heavyweight antidepressant for people who have suffered a major bout of depression and who may have attempted suicide. Manufactured by Pfizer, it's marketed in the UK as Lustral.

As a selective serotonin reuptake inhibitor (SSRI), setraline can be fatal if taken with a monoamine oxidase inhibitor (MAOI). Early warning signs of a likely drug interaction include confusion, irritability and extreme agitation, which leads to delirium and coma, and possibly death. These reactions have also been noticed in people who have recently come off an SSRI and started a MAOI.

You are advised to wait at least 14 days between taking either of these types of drugs.

Similarly, the drug should be prescribed to people with liver disease only with caution, Pfizer advises. Overall, it's designed for short-term use of up to 16 weeks at a daily dosage of 50 mg.

Even without the help of a MAOI, sertraline can pack a punch all on its own. The most common reactions include gastrointestinal complaints, including nausea, diarrhoea, tremors, dizziness, insomnia, sleepiness, sweating, dry mouth and male sexual dysfunction.

In premarketing trials, 15 per cent of the 2,700 patients the drug was tested on had to come off sertraline because of an adverse reaction. Central nervous system disorders come a close second to the gastrointestinal ones in terms of frequency, and included headaches, dizziness and tremors.

Then, of course, there are the paradoxical effects—in other words, it causes the very symptoms it's supposed to treat. Setraline can cause abnormal dreams, aggression, amnesia, delusion, depersonalisation, hallucinations and, yes, depression, aggravated depression and suicidal tendencies.

Reasons to be cheerful indeed.

MANERIX (moclobemide)
Antidepressant

Moclobemide was originally an antituberculosis drug before being developed as an antidepressant, once it was discovered it could produce euphoria in tuberculosis patients.

It is a new-style selective monoamine oxidase inhibitor (MAOI), a class of drugs that supposedly relieves depression by blocking the action of the MAO hormone in the brain. Moclobemide was touted as avoiding many of the well-documented side effects of other MAOIs.

However, experience in Finland suggests that moclobemide may be lethal when taken in combination with other types of antidepressants. Doctors at the University of Helsinki reported five deaths among patients who mixed "moderately low overdoses" of moclobemide with similar doses of other antidepressant drugs (Lancet, 4 December 1993).

In one case, a man of 23 and a woman of 19 took 1,000–1,500 mg of moclobemide along with up to 500 mg of clomipramine, a tricyclic antidepressant (TCA). Two to three hours later, they were euphoric but, within the next two hours, both experienced extreme tremors followed by convulsions and loss of consciousness, said the report. Although they were admitted to hospital, both died between nine to 10 hours after taking the drugs. The researchers say: "Blood concentrations [of both drugs] at admission and necropsy showed only moderate overdosage of these antidepressants."

They also cite the cases of three men who died three to 16 hours after taking overdoses of moclobemide and the selective serotonin reuptake inhibitor (SSRI) citalopram. Their deaths showed a "similar pattern of events" to the two patients who had died from a mixture of MAOI and TCA. "Patients 3 and 4 died despite immediate conventional treatment in hospital."

"Many antidepressants obviously carry a risk of a serious interaction if combined with MAO inhibitors: citalopram, fluoxetine, fluvoxamine, sertraline, and paroxetine are selective inhibitors, but, in addition, clomipramine, trazodone, and imipramine are potent inhibitors of serotonin reuptake." This may mean that patients mixing these and moclobemide could be at risk.

An editorial in the same issue of The Lancet concluded: "Drugs that increase brain serotonin should be given with care."

MAREVAN (warfarin sodium)
Blood-thinning anticoagulant
Warfarin sodium is an anticoagulant, based on vitamin K, which thins the blood to prevent a thrombosis. It may also be prescribed after a heart attack.

But with side effects including bleeding and haemorrhage sometimes resulting in death, it is a treatment that must involve very careful monitoring both by the patient and the doctor.

It is marketed in the US as Coumadin and in the UK as Marevan, among other names.

The manufacturer stresses that the dosage varies from patient to patient, and treatment may have to be stopped, or the dosage reduced, as soon as any reactions, such as bruising, diarrhoea, blood in the stools or fever, occur.

Warfarin can cause haemorrhage from any organ or tissue. Early warning signs include paralysis, headache, chest, abdomen or joint pains, shortness of breath and unexplained swelling. It can also make the toes turn purple, usually after 3–10 weeks of use, which can lead to gangrene unless treated.

It should not be taken by anyone who runs a greater than normal risk of haemorrhage. Pregnant women should never be prescribed the drug not only because of the bleeding risk, but also because warfarin is known to cause malformations of the fetus as well as miscarriage. Breastfeeding mothers should also not take the drug, nor should people low in vitamin C.

The manufacturer considers the elderly as a high-risk group even though they are probably among the most likely to be prescribed the drug.

Special thought also needs to be given if a patient is already taking one of the NSAIDs, such as aspirin.

MEGACE (megestrol)
Breast cancer therapy
If at first tamoxifen doesn't succeed, try, try Megace. That seems to be the policy of many oncologists when they're treating breast cancer.

It may be fashion, it may be because the oncologists see tamoxifen as being a more effective drug but, whatever the reason, Megace seems destined to be always the bridesmaid and never the bride.

In one sense, this collective decision is unfortunate because Megace does not boast anything like the impressive array of side effects and adverse reactions that tamoxifen can muster.

Regular dosage for treating breast cancer is 160 mg a day, and no serious side effects have been detected, even at levels of 1600 mg a day.

But if a drug is to do good, it must also have the potential to do harm, and Megace is no exception.

Pregnant women, in particular, are warned not to take the drug because of the harm it can cause to the fetus. Similarly, breastfeeding mothers should also stop the treatment.

Adverse reactions include weight gain, one of the most common side effects among patients, although this seems to be attributable more to an increased appetite than fluid retention. Though rare, thrombosis is a serious concern, especially among those who may be susceptible.

Other reactions include nausea and vomiting, oedema, bleeding, tumour flare, hyperglycaemia, alopecia (balding), hypertension, carpal tunnel syndrome and rash.

Like so many drugs, Megace seems to have a paradoxical effect when tested on animals. Female dogs developed benign and malignant tumours of the breast after being given the drug for seven years, although these results were not replicated in tests carried out on rats and monkeys.

MINOCIN (minocycline)
Acne treatment

Minocycline has become a first-line treatment in the UK for severe acne. It is also used in the US at specialist skin centres, but its more common use there is to treat infectious diseases.

But how much longer it enjoys this position is in question now that it has been associated with serious adverse reactions, some life-threatening.

Doctors have reported several deaths among patients taking the drug. One 39-year-old woman needed a liver transplant when her liver failed after being on the drug for just four weeks.

Leading US dermatologist Dr Alice Gottlieb wants to see the drug used with greater caution after one study discovered it caused a discoloration of the mouth of 10 per cent of users. Other serious adverse reactions have included autoimmune hepatitis and lupus.

The onset of symptoms have varied. Serum sickness reactions have been reported after just 16 days on the drug, while hypersensitivity reactions, such as rash, fever and liver problems, have been seen within 24 days. Several cases of drug-induced lupus have been reported up to two years.

Minocycline, a tetracycline, is known to cause gastrointestinal problems such as nausea, anorexia, vomiting and diarrhoea.

Tooth discoloration is fairly common, although Wyeth, the manufacturer, says this is reversible once the drug is stopped. Children under the age of 12, whose teeth are still developing, may not be so lucky and may have discoloured teeth for the rest of their lives.

People with a history of liver problems, and pregnant and breastfeeding women, should all avoid the drug.

NEOTIGASON (acitretin)
Psoriasis drug

Acitretin is the generic name of Roche's psoriasis drug, which seems to have got under the skin of the drug regulators. It is also another example to be added to the growing list of drugs that gets an easier passage through the European regulatory framework than the American one.

Acitretin has been available in the UK since the late 1980s, marketed as Neotigason. It is known to cause birth defects, and so must not be prescribed to pregnant women or to those breastfeeding.

Roche had successfully convinced the English regulators that the drug was perfectly safe for women who wanted to become pregnant two years after taking the drug. But then, the company came up against the slightly harder wall of the US Food and Drug Administration.

The drug had been approved in 1996, but had never been marketed when the FDA was asked to take a closer look. Acitretin was promoted as the safer option to etretinate (Tegison), but reports were indicating that acitretin was being metabolised into etretinate in some patients and so had an even higher potential to cause birth defects.

The FDA agreed to change the warning, and increase the period between finishing the drug and conceiving to at least three years. Roche pushed for the European two-year warning, while several members of the evaluating panel wanted to extend the warning for an indefinite period.

As a result, American doctors now have a black-box warning about the drug in their drug reference guide whereas their British equivalents still have to rely on the small print.

Aside from possible birth defects, other adverse reactions include eye problems, headaches, stomachache, tinnitus and sinusitis.

NICOTINELL (nicotine)
Nicotine patches to stop smoking

Nicotinell is one of the leading licensed brands of nicotine patches, used to help people smoking. Introduced in 1992, it is manufactured by Geigy

Pharmaceuticals and has reportedly helped thousands of heavy smokers to quit.

Research from the University Hospital of Wales has concluded that the patches can even help people with ulcerative colitis (N Engl J Med, 24 March 1994).

But some specialists are worried that the patches might become the answer for all smokers when they should be viewed only as a last-resort option for very heavy smokers unable to give up by willpower alone.

Nicotine is a highly toxic drug and doses can be lethal if rapidly absorbed. The patches are intended to leak nicotine into the body once a day; the least powerful patch contains 17.5 mg of nicotine, the middle range has 35 mg and the strongest has 52.5 mg.

People should not smoke when using the patches; five people in the US who did so knowingly to give themselves a nicotine 'rush' died of a heart attack.

Patches should not be used by children—and, indeed, may be fatal to them—nor by pregnant or nursing women, or occasional smokers. Others at risk include those with a heart condition, angina, irregular heart rhythms, skin diseases, ulcers, diabetes, kidney problems and high blood pressure.

Side effects include nausea, vomiting, abdominal pain, diarrhoea, headache, sweating and pallor. The usual litany of problems associated with smoking also applies.

NIVAQUINE (chloroquine)
Malaria drug

A subscriber's fears for her daughter alerted us to chloroquine, which is being prescribed to increasing numbers of travellers who return from even further-flung holidays with malaria. The daughter had recently suffered a fainting fit while on a course of the drug.

As the long list of reactions to chloroquine includes convulsive seizures, we guessed the drug had a part to play. Other common reactions—other than death, which we're coming to—include irreversible eye damage, nerve deafness and tinnitus, anorexia, skin eruptions (and will worsen any psoriasis) and hair loss.

Chloroquine is marketed in the UK as Nivaquine by Rhone-Poulenc and as Avloclor by ICI; in the US, it is available as Aralen Phosphate from Sanofi Winthrop, and as Chloroquine Phosphate tablets by Biocraft.

Chloroquine is not a drug that should be taken lightly, and your own background and health should be carefully considered before it is prescribed.

For the physician, it really is a careful balance between risk and reward.

A number of people have died while on the drug, even when relatively low amounts are taken. One child of three died after being given 0.75 g.

Equally worrying are reports that the drug is no longer effective against some strains of malaria that have become resistant to it, so your doctor may be inclined to increase the recommended dose which, in an adult, is 500 mg once a week.

An early warning sign of a serious adverse reaction is a weakening of the muscles, which should be reported straightaway. The treatment should be stopped immediately.

ORTHO-GYNEST (oestriol)
Postmenopausal vaginal treatment

Ortho-Gynest cream, which contains oestriol, a form of ovarian and placental oestrogen, is often prescribed to perimenopausal women to treat thinning of the vaginal wall or vaginal dryness. Its popularity, to some degree, is due to the fact that doctors see it as being less powerful, and so safer, than HRT.

Nonetheless, the cream's active ingredient is a synthetic, non-steroidal oestrogen. Oestrogens have been linked to endometrial cancer in three independent studies, and the risks of developing endometrial cancer increase by between 4.5 to 13.9 times while women are taking them.

Women who are pregnant or who are thinking of having a baby shouldn't take any oestrogen preparation. There is a strong possibility that oestrogens and progestogens can damage the unborn baby. Indeed, a woman who becomes pregnant while on a course of treatment may be advised by her doctor to seek an abortion.

There are also plenty of hazards in store for the woman who is past her childbearing years. While the link between oestrogens and endometrial cancer seems to be well accepted, there are strong suspicions that oestrogens may also trigger cancer of the breast, cervix, vagina and liver. Women who use the preparation for longer than two years also run the risk of developing gallbladder disease.

Oestrogens also come with all the worries and alarms surrounding the oral contraceptive pill. These adverse reactions include thrombosis, raised blood pressure, glucose intolerance and hypercalcaemia, a condition where there is too much calcium in the blood.

Side effects include fluid retention, depression, *Candida* infections, bleeding, and abdominal cramps or bloating.

transfusions before the patient started to improve (N Engl J Med, 2000; 342: 1773–7).

Researchers point out that ticlopidine had a clean bill of health for seven years before the link with the thrombosis was discovered.

So, as we say, just how safe is safe . . . ?

PONDIMIN (fenfluramine hydrochloride)
Slimming drug

Thousands of obese Americans are on the warpath. They've filed lawsuits claiming they have been injured by taking either Pondimin, Redux or Fen-Phen, all slimming drugs.

The drugs can create lesions or abnormalities in the heart valves, which can result in abnormal blood flow, sometimes causing major health problems.

As the lesions don't usually occur with symptoms, there is no way a patient will know the drug has caused heart damage unless an echocardiogram is carried out. This suggests that the existing lawsuits could be just the tip of a very large iceberg.

American Home Products, the firm responsible for the drug in the US, is "vigorously" disputing the claims, an interesting position as Pondimin (fenfluramine hydrochloride) has a large black-box warning at the beginning of its entry in the *Physicians' Desk Reference*, the American drugs bible. Despite its protestations, the company is planning to voluntarily withdraw the drug from the American market.

The *PDR* warns that the drug can cause cardiac disease, and points to one study which discovered that 24 patients, who were given a combination drug including fenfluramine to treat their obesity, developed heart disease; five needed surgery. Similar cases of heart disease were found in patients taking fenfluramine on its own.

Primary pulmonary hypertension, a rare and often fatal disease, has an "increased frequency" in fenfluramine patients, the *PDR* warning continues. Common reactions include drowsiness and diarrhoea, while other reactions reported include abdominal pain, fever, suicidal tendencies and death.

As well as pulmonary hypertension, other cardiovascular problems that may be seen include heart arrest and failure, heart attack, angina and arrhythmia.

To round things off, asthma, paranoia, speech disorder, vertigo and abnormal thoughts have all been recorded.

But look on the bright side: you don't have to diet.

POSICOR (mibefradil dihydrochloride)
Calcium-channel blocker (heart drug)
The heart drug Posicor (mibefradil dihydrochloride) was withdrawn by the manufacturer after it caused cardiogenic shock in four patients, one of whom died.

The reactions occurred when the patients had another calcium-channel blocker (aka calcium antagonist) added to their prescription.

The patient who died was a 79-year-old woman who started taking nifedipine one day after discontinuing mibefradil. A second woman and a man, both aged 60, both suffered cardiogenic shock within a few hours of starting a new prescription. A fourth woman, aged 55, went into shock within five hours of adding felodipine and enalapril to a regimen that included mibefradil.

The manufacturer, Roche Laboratories, voluntarily withdrew the drug after post-marketing surveillance showed it could lead to serious interactions with the glycoside digoxin and with other calcium antagonists such as verapamil and diltiazem, particularly among elderly patients.

One member of the study team, Michael Mullins, from the Oregon Poison Center, said the drug has a long half-life and that patients should wait at least a week before starting another heart drug like a beta-blocker, and at least two weeks before starting a course of felodipine (a calcium antagonist) or timolol (a beta-blocker).

Strangely, earlier trials had failed to detect any serious adverse reactions. The most common ones—headache, leg oedema and rhinitis—were seen in similar numbers in the placebo group, which left lightheadedness as the only genuine side effect.

This throws into question the current methods of drug testing. Until drugs are tested on the populations for whom they are intended rather than on strapping young students keen to earn extra cash, and reactions with other drugs are more carefully monitored, it's hard to say with any certainty that any drug is 'safe'.

PREMARIN (conjugated oestrogen)
HRT drug
Premarin, a hormone replacement therapy (HRT) drug, is given three pages of closely typed text in the American drugs bible, the *Physicians' Desk Reference* (1995), warning of some of the possible side effects.

Despite these warnings, Premarin is the 23rd best-selling drug in the UK, prescribed mainly to menopausal women.

Manufactured by Wyeth-Ayerst, it is marketed as an antiosteoporosis drug, and is available as a vaginal cream and in tablets.

The direst warnings concern increased risks of developing endometrial cancer with this oestrogen-only preparation, as shown in three independent studies. The risk can increase by nearly 14 times if the drug is taken for more than a year.

Women who are pregnant should not take the drug as limb deformities in the baby may result.

Other possible side effects include cancer of the breast, cervix, vagina and liver (as shown in animals), gallbladder disease, heart attack, stroke, high blood pressure, bleeding, nausea, headaches and weight gain.

If that's not enough to put you off, the way the drug is made might. Mares are placed in very restricted stalls for months on end while their urine is collected. The animals are unable to move more than a few inches in any direction during all that time.

PREPULSID (cisapride)
Dietary aid
Prepulsid joins the growing list of These We Have Loved . . . And Lost. The drug, which speeds food through the stomach, has been withdrawn from the US, British, Canadian and German markets following the high number of deaths associated with the drug.

The American drugs regulator, the Food and Drug Administration, says that 80 people died of heart complications while taking the drug, while another 341 cases of complications have also been reported. Canadian authorities reported a further 10 cases and 44 complications. It was withdrawn from both markets in 2000.

This drug was first brought to our notice a long time before that by an Australian subscriber has alerted us to the side effects of Prepulsid. In the package insert supplied with the drug, the manufacturer Janssen Pharmaceutical says that the drug can cause "mild" abdominal problems.

This was not the experience of our subscriber, however. After taking the correct dosage for two days, she started to suffer mild diarrhoea and flatulence, but this escalated to severe abdominal cramps, which forced her to her bed. "I can assure you that these cramps were not mild; as for my intestines, it felt like a fermentation unit had started up, and it took a month for the resulting flatulence to settle down to a tolerable level. Three months later, I would not describe it as having completely settled down," she writes.

So not only were the cramps not mild, they were also far from transitory.

Her doctor confirmed that Prepulsid was the likely cause.

Needless to say, she came off the treatment immediately. By doing so, she avoided some of the other side effects listed in *The Data Sheet Compendium* (now *The Medicines Compendium*). These include headaches, lightheadedness and, more rarely, convulsions.

For those who are particularly unfortunate, liver function abnormalities have been reported, although no direct link to the drug has been proven.

Children under the age of 12, pregnant women and people with liver or kidney problems should not be given the drug. Normal dosage is three 10-mg tablets three times a day.

Prepulsid is one example of a growing number of cases that show up the inadequacies of the licensing process, which allows lethal drugs such as this onto the market in the first place.

PROSCAR (finasteride)
Benign prostate treatment

Proscar (finasteride) quickly established itself as the treatment of choice for benign enlarged prostate in the US and the UK.

But its status was thrown into question by a study conducted by the University of Washington which showed that finasteride is no more effective than a sugar pill. Researchers tracked 1,229 patients, aged between 45 and 80, for a year to see if the drug was effective compared with terazosin, an alpha-blocker, and a placebo. They found no difference between finasteride and placebo in terms of quality of life measures.

This finding is contrary to an earlier trial showing that the drug was very effective in reducing the prostate over a year. But the earlier trial apparently involved men with larger prostates whereas those in the University of Washington survey had prostates of a size found more generally "in the real world," as research team leader Professor Michael Brawer put it.

All of this may be bad news for earlier finasteride patients who suffered from any one of the side effects that come with the drug, including impotence, reduced sexual interest, breast tenderness and enlargement, and hypersensitivity reactions such as lip swelling and skin rashes.

These reactions have been observed among patients taking the standard, recommended dose of 5 mg a day. In tests on mice, death has occurred with single dosages of 1500 mg.

One piece of good news for prostate sufferers: the Washington study did find that terazosin was very effective in treating patients with 'normally' enlarged prostates. Improvements were noted within two weeks.

PROZAC (fluoxetine)

Antidepressant

Prozac (fluoxetine) was introduced by Eli Lilly in 1987 as a safer kind of antidepressant. Experience, however, suggests that far from being safer, Prozac may be highly dangerous to the person taking the tablets and to those in his or her immediate vicinity.

In the US, Eli Lilly has been facing more than 100 civil lawsuits from people claiming that Prozac led them to suicidal and violent thoughts and actions.

In some cases, the level of violence involved is horrific: one man shot and killed eight people at his workplace and injured a dozen others before killing himself; a woman attacked her mother, biting her more than 20 times, leaving bite-sized pieces of flesh on the floor.

Despite growing concern, the US Food and Drug Administration decided in 1991 that there was no evidence that Prozac had been instrumental in the violence. Writing in Townsend Letter for Doctors (February/March 1993), however, medical investigative reporter Gary Null points out that everyone on the FDA committee had a vested interest in giving the drug a clean bill of health and so refused to consider vital evidence being put forward by critics of Prozac.

In the UK, Ian Oswald wrote to the British Medical Journal (26 October 1991) to point out that a supposedly impartial report vindicating Prozac that the journal had published earlier (BMJ, 21 September 1991) was anything but independent.

"At a time when the manufacturer is facing litigation, the corporate defence attorneys will be pleased by the journal having published a piece authored wholly by the manufacturer's employees," he commented dryly.

Leaving aside the odd alleged murderous rampage, other side effects associated with Prozac are disorders of the nervous system, such as tardive dystonia, where the muscles involuntarily twitch or go into spasm, anxiety, nervousness and insomnia, anorexia, seizures, severe skin rashes and vasculitis, a potentially fatal inflammation of the blood vessels.

PULMICORT (budesonide)

Steroid for childhood asthma

Not content with injecting live vaccines into the immature immune systems of babies, the medical authorities have recently approved the use of a steroid for tots just three months old.

The news has already been welcomed with unquestioningly open arms in some quarters. The English arch-advocate of all things orthodox, Dr Thomas Stuttaford, believes that Pulmicort (budesonide) could be as important to the modern mum as gripe water was to her mother and grandmother.

Pulmicort, made by Astra, is an inhaler designed to relieve asthma and croup. It is the first product for croup to receive British approval, and can be given to children as young as three months, says the manufacturer.

Dr Stuttaford says that, as a steroid, it has few—if any—side effects, which may come as a surprise to those claiming damage from steroids.

The statement may come as a bit of a surprise to the manufacturer, too. It warns that the drug may cause sudden bronchoconstriction as well as throat irritation, coughing and hoarseness.

According to the listed side effects of another version of the generic budesonide, also manufactured by Astra, it suppresses the immune system so that normally innocuous diseases such as chickenpox and measles may become killers, a point worth checking if your child is on the drug and is about to have his first innoculations.

Perhaps, then, not quite so benign as gripe water after all.

PUMPHEP (heparin)
Anticoagulant for heart patients

Heparin (the generic name for a range of drugs, including HepLok in the US, and PumpHep and Unihep in the UK) is an anticoagulant that is often used as a just-in-case therapy if there is a danger of heart attack or stroke. It is also used to prevent blood clots.

Its most common side effect is haemorrhage. Because bleeding can occur at virtually any part of the body, it should not be given to those who are at an increased risk of haemorrhage, such as those suffering from peptic ulcers, bacterial heart infection and even during menstruation. Women over 60 are also at greater risk.

Extensive reviews of the available literature show that much depends on the dose and method of administration, and whether or not it is given in conjunction with other drugs, particularly antiplatelet drugs like aspirin. Heparin is generally given either as a subcutaneous injection or an intra-venous infusion. Some patients experience local irritation following deep, subcutaneous injections. Intramuscular injections are not recommended as they seem to have the highest rate of complications, such as skin irritation, ulceration, haematoma and mild pain.

When heparin is given with aspirin, the risk of haemorrhage increases and some of the most serious complications, such as adrenal and ovarian

LIST OF DRUGS

haemorrhage, may be difficult to detect. It has also been shown to result in osteoporosis.

Among the most dramatic side effects of heparin use is 'white clot syndrome' or recurrent thrombosis, which can affect as many as 30 per cent of patients, according to the *Physicians' Desk Reference*. This can lead to skin necrosis, gangrene leading to amputation, heart failure, pulmonary embolism, stroke and even death.

QUESTRAN (cholestyramine)
Cholesterol-lowering drug
Questran is one of a host of drugs routinely prescribed to lower supposedly raised cholesterol levels in patients.

Prescriptions of cholesterol-lowering drugs are generally on the up-and-up. But one study (BMJ, 22 May 1993) suggests that, at best, the numbers of people likely to be helped by these drugs are small. Only those "at very high initial risk of coronary heart disease" were likely to benefit; for those at medium risk, the drugs made no difference; and those at low risk were more likely to die if treated. Quite simply, cholesterol-lowering drugs may reduce your risk of heart attack, but you are more likely to die instead from cancer, respiratory disease, trauma and digestive diseases. (Such deaths are not, however, seen when cholesterol is lowered by changes in diet.)

No association has been proved between supposedly high cholesterol levels in women and heart disease, something which "reinforces doubts about the wisdom of extrapolating results derived from high-risk, middle-aged men to the female population", according to the BMJ.

Side effects specific to Questran (cholestyramine) include constipation, flatulence, heartburn, nausea, diarrhoea, stomach upsets, skin rashes and, rarely, fat in the faeces. It can also lead to vitamin K deficiency, which may cause increased bleeding due to the inability of the blood to clot properly. In animal studies, cholestyramine has been shown to cause intestinal cancer.

RAPAMUNE (sirolimus)
Immunosuppressant after organ transplants
The subtle hand of the pharmaceutical company touches many things, influencing many people such as journalists, researchers and academics. Sometimes 'independent' books are entirely funded by a drug company, and nobody is any the wiser. That is, until something goes wrong.

America's health professionals recently received a free copy of a book that extolled the virtues of Rapamune (sirolimus) as an immunosuppressant for liver transplants. The book was funded by an "unrestricted educational grant" from Wyeth, the manufacturer of Rapamune.

Unfortunately, the authors were overzealous in their praise of the drug. In fact, in trials where the drug had been used with liver transplants, the patient had sometimes died within 30 days.

Wyeth pulled the drug from liver transplant trials after initial findings went against it. In one, over 5 per cent of the liver transplant patients suffered blood clots within 16 days of transplantation while on the drug compared with 0.9 per cent in those taking the immunosuppressant tacrolimus. In another, 8.9 per cent of Rapamune patients suffered a thrombosis compared with 3.8 per cent of tacrolimus patients.

It's not the first time the drug has come to the attention of the health authorities. Wyeth has also been taken to task over the labelling on the packaging that so confused several nurses that they gave the wrong dosage to six people, including a child.

Rapamune was originally intended to stop organ rejection in kidney transplant patients, and is meant to be taken with cyclosporin and corticosteroids. Aside from the occasional death, Rapamune can also raise your cholesterol and triglyceride levels, and cause high blood pressure, anaemia, acne, rash, joint pain and diarrhoea, and decrease your potassium and blood platelet levels.

RELENZA (zanamivir)
Influenza treatment
It's one thing to get a drug approved for use; it's quite another for the National Health Service to agree to adopt it.

GlaxoWellcome found this out to its cost after it developed Relenza (zanamivir), the first drug for treating influenza. The stumbling block proved to be the National Institute for Clinical Excellence (NICE), which assesses for the NHS the effectiveness and cost-effectiveness of drugs and treatments. It found the drug wanting on both counts on reviewing it in October 1999. NICE felt that there wasn't enough research to suggest that 'at-risk' patients—people over 65 or with an existing condition that might make influenza a more serious problem—would benefit from the drug.

Separately, the US Food and Drug Administration (FDA) also noted that wheezing had occurred in some patients with mild-to- moderate asthma after taking the drug.

At £24 for a five-day course of treatment, the drug would cost the NHS up to £15 million a year if there was a flu epidemic.

Thirteen months later, NICE said the drug can be prescribed to people at risk. NICE also said that further analysis suggests that the drug reduces symptoms among the 'at-risk' group by 1.2 days and that, overall, it reduces the risk of complications by 6 per cent.

But there was one important dissenting voice. The editor of the Drug and Therapeutics Bulletin, Professor Joe Collier, who was part of the NICE committee that assessed zanamivir, believed a wrong decision was made.

The Bulletin maintained that the study was flawed and did not focus on 'at-risk' patients, as NICE believes. Even if it did, the fact that it reduced the duration of symptoms by one day is hardly compelling, and nobody has tested the drug against over-the-counter remedies such as paracetamol (acetaminophen) and ibuprofen.

NICE also did not touch upon the increased risk of bronchospasm, particularly among patients with asthma or chronic pulmonary disease.

All of which leaves the health professional with a dilemma to be cautious or NICE.

RELPAX (eletriptan)
Migraine treatment

Eletriptan is one of the newer breed of 'triptans' for treating migraine, following in the wake of the more famous sumatriptan. It's cheaper and is more effective than oral sumatriptan—and a recent major trial reports that it also comes with similar adverse reactions.

The triptan family tries to control migraine attacks by changing serotonin (5-HT) levels, which also affect depression and psychosis.

However, their effectiveness can be hit-or-miss as they are poorly absorbed by the gut. As a result, only around two-thirds of patients are ever helped by the triptans. Even the later injected triptans have a relatively high failure rate, and are also much more expensive. The injected variety of sumatriptan also comes with more adverse reactions.

The triptans are no-go drugs for people suffering from a heart condition as they can cause chest pains in up to 8 per cent of patients.

The later triptans, including eletriptan, naratriptan and rizatriptan, were supposed to come without the reactions associated with sumatriptan. But a study of eletriptan suggests that it has all the usual side effects (Neurology 2000; 54: 156–63).

Flushing, palpitations, nasal discomfort, eye irritation, visual disturbance and agitation were symptoms reported way above those in the placebo group.

In a critique of triptans by Nicholas Bateman of the Scottish Poisons

Information Bureau, there seems little to choose between them (Lancet, 2000; 355: 860–1). Naratriptan seems to have fewer adverse reactions, but also acts more slowly.

A better agent for treating migraine is still needed, he believes, especially as regular use of any of the triptans can produce an increase in migraine frequency and symptoms (Lancet, 1999; 353: 378).

Which, as Hamlet might have said, is a real bummer.

RETIN-A (tretinoin)
Acne therapy
Retin-A is the brand name both in the UK and the US for tretinoin, originally developed to treat acne. As such (and because of its largely disputed claim to eliminate wrinkles), it is among the 50 best-selling drugs in the US.

Manufactured by Ortho, it is available as a lotion, gel or cream; the lotion is best suited for large areas, such as the back, the gel for severe cases of acne, and the cream for dry and fair skin.

It is a very powerful treatment, although the manufacturer is not exactly sure how it works. With it comes a range of side effects that, so far, have all been reversible. The most common is severe rash and peeling, an indication that the treatment should be suspended or stopped.

The treatment should not be used by eczema sufferers, or by pregnant women and those who are breastfeeding. Although there has never been a study in pregnant women, Retin-A has been found to affect fetal growth in rats. "Tretinoin should be used during pregnancy only if the potential benefit justifies the potential risk to the fetus," says the US *Physicians' Desk Reference* (1992) although, as we are talking about acne, it's hard to imagine an instance when that would apply.

Equally worrying are the potential risks that Retin-A users can run when out in the sun. The manufacturer has made it very clear that people should not be exposed to sunlight for any length of time, or use sunlamps while using the treatment. Those with suntans should wait for normal colouring to return before using the drug.

The worry is about the possible link to skin cancer, although no long-term studies, either in humans or animals, have ever been carried out. Small-scale tests among animals have produced varying results.

REZULIN (troglitazone)
Drug for type II diabetes
Drug regulators and, indeed, pharmaceutical companies themselves, often

reassure themselves that the patient knows the risks of the drug he is taking because of the insert provided with each packet. Small print, perhaps, but it's all there if you have the mind, and a magnifying glass, to read it.

But is the whole truth printed on the inserts? Doubts have been raised following a review of a new class of drugs called thiazolidinediones, designed to treat type II diabetes.

Rezulin (troglitazone) was one of the first to be licensed both in the UK and the USA—and was voluntarily withdrawn after it had been linked to a number of liver-poisoning deaths. In America, at least 63 patients died while using the drug, and many more who suffered are filing class-action lawsuits against the manufacturer.

They claim the drug company downplayed the risks, which were first drawn to the public's attention by a study carried out by the Institute of Molecular and Cellular Genetics and Biology in Illkirch, France. It found that 2 per cent of patients suffer hepatic dysfunction, which can lead to liver failure, a potentially lethal side effect not noted by the drug company (Lancet, 2000; 355: 1008–10).

Not surprising, really, says Sidney Wolfe of the Public Citizen's Health Research Group. Only one of 11 efficacy studies for two other thiazolidinediones submitted to the US Food and Drug Administration as part of the approval packages has been published (Lancet, 2000; 356: 254).

His own research into FDA data sources has also revealed that thiazolidinediones can lead to heart failure, "a serious finding not previously adequately acknowledged in the product labelling or on the company websites," he states.

Reactions that the drug company does accept include infections, headache, pain, dizziness, nausea, rhinitis, diarrhoea and urinary tract infections.

Less common is jaundice, but this is reversed once the patients are taken off the drug. Even without liver and heart failure, perhaps even the small print that is published might give a potential patient pause.

RIFATER (isoniazid)
Tuberculosis drug
The risk–benefit balance is always a delicate one in medicine: simply put, are the risks associated with a drug or treatment outweighed by its potential to prevent illness or ease pain?

Such is the dilemma facing a group of parents whose children attend a nursery in South London, where there was an outbreak of TB.

Health officials want to put the children on a six-month regime of the antituberculosis drug Rifater (isoniazid). Unfortunately, in medicine, it's usually the case that the crueller the disease, the crueller the drug, and that is certainly the case with isoniazid.

In the *Physicians' Desk Reference*, the US drugs bible, isoniazid earns a special black-box warning because it can lead to severe and sometimes fatal hepatitis. On the face of it, there is no need to worry overmuch, as cases thus far recorded indicate that such a severe reaction is age-related.

No cases have been reported in the 0–20 age range whereas eight cases per 1,000 have been recorded among the over-65s who have taken the drug. However, delving around 3,000 words on, we discover that "safety and effectiveness in children or adolescents under the age of 15 have not been established". This means that, as is usually the case, the drug has never been tested on children in a controlled clinical trial.

As a result, we don't actually know if it works on children or what might happen if they take it. Seeing this, many a GP may have only rarely, if at all, prescribed isoniazid to a small child.

This may explain why zero cases of fatal hepatitis have been reported among the under-20s. So the issue of danger may not, after all, be age-related, but simply dose-related. Zero cases have been reported because zero numbers have been taking it.

The problem is that health officials can hide behind spurious statistics such as these to support a decision and convince a worried parent. Of course, his heart may well be in the right place—in this case, he's trying to stop an outbreak of TB—but is that justification enough?

And has the risk–benefit ratio really been proven?

RITALIN (methylphenidate)
Amphetamine for hyperactive children
Ritalin (methylphenidate), taken by as many as a million American children to control attention-deficit and hyperactivity disorder (ADHD, or ADD), has been largely resisted by parents in Britain—until recently. Lately, much media attention has been focused on Ritalin as a drug that can 'unlock' a child's potential compared with the supposed limitations of the dietary approach to hyperactivity.

The view espoused by Ritalin promoters is that the drug, an amphetamine, works by correcting biochemical imbalances in the brain. Not only is there no evidence to support that view, but there's no evidence to suggest that

Ritalin makes any lasting change. As the manufacturer Ciba admits in the *Physicians' Desk Reference*, there are no long-term studies on safety and effectiveness. Furthermore, *The American Textbook of Psychiatry* shows a 75 per cent improvement with Ritalin compared with a 40 per cent response with a placebo, suggesting that half the response to Ritalin could be purely down to the 'placebo effect', where the belief that a drug will work seems to improve symptoms.

What we do know is that Ritalin suppresses growth, makes a child more prone to seizures, and causes visual disturbances, nervousness, insomnia, anorexia and toxic psychosis. It's worth remembering that this drug is a class II-category controlled substance, like barbiturates, morphine and others with a high potential for addiction or abuse. Uppers supposedly have a paradoxical effect on children, quieting them down, but often the effect is mixed. Children are subdued during the day, but stimulated at night and thus unable to sleep. The *PDR* entry for the drug carries a special black-box warning of drug dependence and psychotic episodes: "Careful supervision is required during drug withdrawal, since severe depression as well as the effects of chronic overactivity can be unmasked".

Numerous cases of suicide after drug withdrawal have been reported. One study (J Am Acad Child Adolesc Psychiatry, 1987; 26: 56–64) showed that children treated only with stimulants (rather than drugs and counselling) had higher arrest records and were more likely to be institutionalised.

Peter Breggin, author of *Toxic Psychiatry* (HarperCollins, 1991), notes that long-term use causes irritability and hyperactivity—the very problems the drug is supposed to treat. One study showed evidence of brain atrophy in more than half of 24 adults treated with psychostimulants (Psychiatr Res, 1986: 245). In another study in Johannesburg involving 14 children, only two responded to the drug (South Afr Med J, 17 Sept 1988). One child showed "significant" deterioration, and another "marked" deterioration.

ROACCUTANE (isotretinoin)
Acne treatment

How long does it take for a drug regulator to act after receiving alarming reports from doctors about a drug? A few weeks? Perhaps a few months? How about seven years.

That is the time it has taken the US drugs regulator, the Food and Drug Administration (FDA), to respond to reports on the acne drug Roaccutane (isotretinoin), marketed in the US as Accutane.

Concerns about the drug were first raised in Australia in 1993, after a woman gave birth to a severely malformed baby. She had been using the drug before conception and for the first five weeks of gestation.

This soon became such a concern that the manufacturer tried to educate users to take contraception before starting the drug. Despite this, a large number of babies in the womb were put at risk because women started the treatment while pregnant. And doctors were blissfully prescribing the drug when they really should have known better.

The drug has also caused miscarriage, premature birth and death of the infant. The Center for Drug Evaluation and Research in the US says that "there is an extremely high risk that a baby will be deformed or will die" if the patient is pregnant when taking the drug.

Another concern is that the drug may trigger depression and other serious mental problems, including suicidal thoughts. Some patients have actually taken their own lives.

So, finally, the FDA has decided to act. It has issued a letter to all health practitioners, alerting them to the dangers. It is also changing the warning on the product label. All this after seven years of reports of something being seriously wrong.

Now all we have to do is get the doctor to read it.

ROFERON-A (interferon)
Powerful anticancer drug

Roferon-A is a neutron bomb of a drug designed to megablast the most pernicious of systemic conditions, but not necessarily to leave the patient standing. As such, it won the accolade in the UK of becoming the first approved treatment for chronic hepatitis C.

Not that its earlier targets were any less ambitious. It was designed by its manufacturer Roche to treat hairy cell leukaemia and AIDS-related Kaposi's sarcoma, and is based on the generic interferon alpha-2a.

It is given by injection and, naturally, only under medical supervision. As an anticancer drug, it is able to slow the growth of tumours, although researchers admit they do not know how it does this which, in itself, is a worry.

Adverse reactions are better understood. As risks tend to rise in relation to benefits, and as Roferon-A is treating life-threatening conditions, it almost goes without saying that reactions can be severe, and include death itself.

You, the patient, should be warned of these risks beforehand. And if you are under 18 (an X-rated drug?), have a history of heart or kidney disease, seizures or a compromised central nervous system, this drug is not for you.

Reactions can include a heart attack, albeit rarely, but more common are those relating to the central nervous system, such as decreased mental function, depression, insomnia, dizziness and even coma.

Virtually all patients suffer some flu-like symptom, and other possible reactions include a skin rash, vertigo, muscle contractions, earache, eye irritations, tremor and, believe it or not, hepatitis.

Daily dosages for hairy cell leukaemia are 3 million IU and, for Kaposi's sarcoma, 36 million IU. Dosages should not be altered, nor should the patient use different varieties of interferon during a course.

If your doctor allows you to administer the drug yourself, make sure you are well hydrated and understand all the rules of needle use.

ROXIAM (remoxipride)
Antipsychotic

Remoxipride is an antipsychotic drug, marketed as Roxiam in the UK by Astra Pharmaceuticals. It is used to treat schizophrenia and other forms of psychoses that are accompanied by delusions, hallucinations and thought disorders, and is claimed to have fewer extrapyramidal (involuntary movement) side effects than other antipsychotics.

However, some worrying complications are emerging which don't appear to have been discovered in the drug's earlier premarketing trials. Towards the end of 1993, the UK Committee on Safety of Medicines, the body that monitors the safety of drugs in circulation, issued a warning that there had been eight reports of aplastic anaemia from among 50,000 patients using remoxipride worldwide. Aplastic anaemia is a potentially fatal deficiency of blood cells caused by a failure of the cell-producing mechanisms in bone marrow.

The CSM warning was followed by a report from doctors at the Department of Haematology and Pharmacy at the UK's Leicester Royal Infirmary of a 63-year-old schizophrenic who developed red cell aplasia (anaemia with normal bone marrow) and thrombocytopenia (lower than normal blood platelets, resulting in bleeding and easy bruising) after daily doses of 600 mg of remoxipride for a year (Lancet, 5 February 1994).

This case, together with the earlier reports, led the Leicester doctors to conclude: "Patients on remoxipride therapy may be at risk of developing severe blood [abnormalities] and require careful monitoring."

According to *The Data Sheet Compendium* (now *The Medicines Compendium*), other effects of remoxipride include insomnia, anxiety, aggressiveness, nausea and headache. It can also cause muscle spasms.

SANDIMMUN (cyclosporin)
Immunosuppressant for psoriasis
Cyclosporin (cyclosporine in the US)—or Sandimmun (Sandimmune in the US)—is a classic example of a drug being developed for one use, then 'borrowed' for the treatment of other, unrelated, conditions. This powerful immunosuppressant was originally developed for organ transplants: by suppressing the immune system, it makes it less likely that a donated organ will be identified and rejected as being, literally, a 'foreign body'.

Now, however, cyclosporin is beginning to be used for many conditions such as psoriasis that are thought to be triggered by an oversensitive immune-system response.

Not surprisingly, for a potent drug developed for use in the extreme situation of a transplant, cyclosporin brings with it a whole host of dangerous side effects. It has been shown to be effective for difficult-to-treat cases of psoriasis (N Engl J Med, 31 January 1991), but those patients may be merely swapping one severe, but non-life-threatening, skin condition for another that is far worse—skin cancer. It has been shown to cause other types of malignancies as well, including lymphoma (cancer of the lymph nodes, thymus, tonsils and spleen).

It is also associated with liver and kidney damage. The American *Physicians' Desk Reference* warns that, of those transplant patients receiving cyclosporin who suffer kidney damage as a result, "from 5 per cent to 10 per cent . . . will fail to show a deduction in a rising serum creatinine [a waste product of the body's metabolism] despite a decrease or discontinuation of cyclosporine therapy." In other words, the damage to kidneys is permanent.

Inevitably, because cyclosporin suppresses the immune system, the body becomes more susceptible to infections. There have also been reports of adults and children suffering convulsions while taking the drug. And one in 1,000 patients has experienced anaphylactic reactions, including flushing of the face and chest, acute respiratory distress and wheezing, rapid pulse rate and high blood pressure.

SEPTRIN (trimethoprim)
Antibacterial
Septrin is an antibacterial drug used to treat everything from traveller's diarrhoea to HIV infection. As a sulphonamide drug, it has a particularly bizarre pedigree, originating from the dye industry in the 1930s when it was discovered that dye products had antibacterial properties.

It is an extremely toxic drug. The US *Physicians' Desk Reference* carries a warning in bold capital letters: "FATALITIES ASSOCIATED WITH THE ADMINISTRATION OF SULFONAMIDES, ALTHOUGH RARE, HAVE OCCURRED DUE TO SEVERE REACTIONS." These reactions include Stevens–Johnson syndrome (a disorder of the skin and mucous membranes characterised by swelling, blistering and ulcers), hepatic necrolysis (death of liver tissue), agranulocytosis (low white blood cells), anaemia, other blood disorders and hypersensitivity of the respiratory tract. These are symptoms that have been associated with HIV, but which may, in fact, be drug-induced.

Apparently trivial reactions, like skin rashes, sore throat or cough, may be early indications of something more serious and potentially fatal, it warns. The *PDR* also recommends that, because of the likelihood of severe blood disorders, complete blood counts should be done frequently. And, of course, the drug should be stopped at the first sign of any side effect.

Septrin's most common adverse effects include gastrointestinal disturbances such as nausea, vomiting and anorexia (symptoms similar to the traveller's diarrhoea it may be being used to treat), and allergic reactions such as rashes and hives.

AIDS patients being treated with the drug for *Pneumocystis carinii* pneumonia (PCP), an opportunistic infection associated with AIDS, have a "greatly increased" likelihood of suffering side effects compared with non-AIDS patients, says the *PDR*. The shopping list of other reactions includes hepatitis, kidney failure, eye problems, inability to pass urine, abdominal pain, aseptic meningitis, convulsions, tinnitus (ringing in the ears), hallucinations and depression, to name but a few.

SERETIDE (fluticasone propionate)
Asthma treatment
There's a wind of change in asthma treatment, or certainly as far as the marketing men are concerned. They've been sharpening their pencils to tell doctors about Seretide, a new asthma inhaler designed for sufferers who are not getting relief from low-to-moderate doses of inhaled steroids.

Best of all, they continue, the patient is likely to enjoy improvements from the very first day "which may aid compliance"—doctor-speak for saying the patient will be a good boy and will continue taking the treatment. And at a cost to the NHS of nearly £67 for one pack of Seretide 500, that's pretty important.

For "wind of change", read "wind of haven't we seen this before somewhere", but of course, that doesn't read quite as well. Seretide is a combination of two established GlaxoWellcome asthma inhalers: salmeterol and fluticasone propionate, marketed respectively as Serevent and Flovent.

There's no way of knowing just how new Seretid compares with the combined drugs from which it has sprung, but it comes with its own bundle of side effects, some of which are shared with its parents. Typical reactions can include oral candidiasis, hoarseness, throat irritation, headache, palpitations, hypersensitivity, tremor, irregular heart rhythms, myalgia and muscle cramps.

Like most drugs, Seretide can also have a paradoxical effect: in other words, it may cause the very symptoms it's supposed to be treating. And like other steroids, it can also cause growth retardation in adolescents, reduce bone mineral density or cause eye problems such as cataract or glaucoma.

So, if doctors do decide to introduce a wind of change into their asthma therapy, it looks as though they'll need to monitor their patients with great care or run the risk of reaping the whirlwind.

SEREVENT (salmeterol xinafoate)
Asthma inhaler

"I sleep well" is the headline used to market Allen & Hanburys' antiasthma inhaler Serevent. Such a statement may be just a dream for many users; tests have shown that up to 28 per cent suffer headaches while on the drug, and 14 per cent may develop an upper respiratory tract infection.

Other reactions reported by the test group included palpitations, laryngitis, nausea, vomiting, dental pain, back and joint pain, cramping, fatigue, bronchitis, rash and skin eruptions. If those aren't enough to cause sleepless nights, you also might like to know that Serevent includes ozone-destroying chemicals.

Like so many other drugs, Serevent also has the paradoxical effect of causing brochospasms, the very thing it is supposedly treating.

Serevent is designed as a supplementary treatment for those who need added relief from asthma at night, or if they suffer brochospasms after exercise.

Standard dosage is 42 mcg twice a day; the manufacturer stresses that doses should be at least 12 hours apart. Not surprisingly, tests have shown that some of the reactions, most noticeably tremors, nervousness and palpitations, increase with the dose.

Those who should not take the drug include pregnant women, possibly those who are nursing, although there is no absolute evidence on this, and the elderly should be carefully monitored while on the drug, especially if they are suffering some heart condition. Anyone with liver problems should not take the drug because it may accumulate in blood plasma if the body cannot dispel it.

SEROXAT (paroxetine hydrochloride)
SSRI antidepressant

Seroxat (paroxetine hydrochloride) is an antidepressant that has been causing concern to the UK's Committee on Safety of Medicines. Manufactured by SmithKline Beecham, it is part of the SSRI (selective serotonin reuptake inhibitor) family that also includes Prozac.

It's been suspected of causing six cases of hepatitis in the UK, although only two were subsequently confirmed by biopsy.

Nonetheless, liver damage has been frequently linked to the drug, and 54 cases have been reported to the Committee on Safety of Medicines.

The drug might also cause the eye disease glaucoma, as happened with one 84-year-old woman.

Taking any SSRI with a monoamine oxidase inhibitor (MAOI) can be lethal. Mixing the two drugs can trigger hyperthermia and sudden changes in mental states that can lead to delirium and coma.

But the SSRIs can cause damage without the assistance of another drug. In tests, the drug was found to bring on mania attacks, seizures, suicidal tendencies and abnormal bleeding.

Overall, up to 20 per cent of people suffering from depression have to stop taking the drug because of some adverse reaction, such as insomnia, agitation, tremors, anxiety, dizziness, constipation, nausea, diarrhoea, vomiting, impotence and sweating.

The figure falls to around 12 per cent in patients taking the drug for panic attacks or obsessive/compulsive disorders.

Over one-quarter of all patients will suffer nausea while on the drug, the most common reaction, noted in 26 per cent of all users. This is followed by drowsiness (23 per cent), headache and dry mouth (both 18 per cent).

The manufacturer has been ordered by America's drug regulator, the Food and Drug Administration, to strengthen its warning about sudden withdrawal of the drug. Instead, the dose should be reduced gradually. The move follows action from around 60 patients in Britain who suffered severe reactions after suddenly coming off the drug.

The manufacturer was also in breach of the international pharmaceutical code of practice when it claimed on American television that no patient had suffered from a sudden withdrawal of the drug.

SPORANOX (itraconazole)
Antifungal treatment

Sporanox (itraconazole) is an antifungal that packs a punch. In the US, three cases of reversible hepatitis were discovered among 2,500 people taking part in the first trials, and another patient outside of the US died but, as he was taking various medications, the precise cause of death cannot be identified.

But if Sporanox is potent, it can be lethal when taken in conjunction with the antihistamine terfenadine. One person died while on the dual medication, and three cases of life-threatening irregular heartbeat were also reported.

In another test in the US, 10.6 per cent of the patients had to come off the drug because of adverse reactions mainly associated with gastrointestinal disorders, such as nausea, vomiting and diarrhoea. Nearly 9 per cent reported a skin rash, while headache and raised blood pressure were also common complaints. Nearly 3 per cent reported liver problems.

The American drugs regulator, the Food and Drug Administration, has issued a warning about the drug, pointing out its association to congestive heart failure and liver reactions. Between 1992 and 2001, it is thought that around 13 patients died from congestive heart failure while on the drug.

This range of reactions seems a high price to pay for a drug that's supposed to treat conditions that mainly cause discomfort, such as candidiasis, thrush and other fungal infections, such as of the fingernails.

Manufactured by Janssen-Cilag, Sporanox comes in 100-mg capsules, and the dosage varies widely depending on the infection and the condition of the patient. AIDS sufferers, for instance, are supposed to be given double the dose because of their absorption problems.

Patients who show early signs of possible liver problems, unusual fatigue, anorexia, nausea, vomiting and jaundice should come off the drug immediately for tests.

Pregnant women, nursing mothers, children and the elderly should not be given the drug.

TEGRETOL (carbamazepine)
Analgesic for neuralgia

Tegretol (carbamazepine) is an anticonvulsant and analgesic for neuralgia that comes with its fair share of adverse reactions. Doctors in Holland have just found one more to add to the list.

They have discovered that the symptoms of multiple sclerosis (MS) patients are considerably worsened if they are given even low doses of the drug (BMJ, 2000; 320: 1113).

A 48-year-old patient was unable to walk after starting carbamazepine, but strength returned to his legs within two days of the treatment being stopped. In a second case, a 67-year-old woman suffered a similar reaction, although doctors at first assumed that it was a worsening of her MS.

The major worry about the drug, however, is that it might trigger aplastic anaemia and agranulocytosis; people on the drug are eight times more likely to develop one of these conditions. You might also suffer a sudden drop in platelet or white blood cell counts.

Tegretol has also been linked to skin disorders which, while rare, have sometimes been fatal. Other reactions have included congestive heart failure, impotence, hallucinations, vomiting, conjunctivitis, aseptic meningitis and anorexia.

Patients are advised to take a crash-course in identifying early signs of a blood problem, such as fever, sore throat, rashes, ulcers and easy bruising, before starting the drug. If any of these symptoms arise, the patient is urged to visit the doctor immediately. Dizziness and drowsiness may follow, so it is wiser to take a taxi rather than drive yourself.

Tegretol should not be given to anyone with a history of bone marrow depression, and a patient with any blood disorder could also suffer a serious reaction. The MS sufferer can now be added to this long list.

TICLID (ticlopidine hydrochloride)
Antistroke therapy

There seems to be growing interest in Ticlid (ticlopidine hydrochloride), which is designed to reduce the risk of stroke among patients at risk.

In America, Geneva Pharmaceuticals, the distributor of Ticlid, has issued a 'Dear Doctor' letter but, significantly, has addressed it to "Dear concerned health professional".

The concern seems to be caused by the large number of side effects, including severe and fatal blood disorders that the drug can cause. The most dangerous is the sudden drop in the white blood cell count, a condition called neutropenia, which early trials indicated could affect around 2.4 per cent of patients.

Ticlid is, in any event, only supposed to be given to those who cannot tolerate aspirin, but Geneva Pharmaceuticals is now advising doctors to first screen patients for any possible adverse reaction before prescribing.

As Ticlid causes an adverse reaction in 60 per cent of all users, the chances of it being prescribed have probably just dropped dramatically. The most common reaction is diarrhoea, which affects more than 12 per cent of patients, followed by nausea and dyspepsia (both 7 per cent), while over 5 per cent develop a rash.

Rarer, but more serious, conditions caused by the drug include anaemia, hepatitis, kidney failure and lupus.

But the most worrying side effect seems to be neutropenia. It can often be fatal if undetected and untreated, because it lowers the body's natural resistance to disease. The drug's manufacturer Roche Laboratories urges doctors to test the blood of the patient every fortnight for the first three months, the time when neutropenia is most likely to occur.

And, concludes Geneva Pharmaceutical's letter, if your patient does die, please tell the authorities. OK?

TRILUDAN (terfenadine)
Antihistamine for hayfever

Terfenadine, the antihistamine designed to treat hayfever and other allergic reactions, is in the category of These We Have Loved . . . But Lost. The American drugs regulator, the Food and Drug Administration (FDA), withdrew the drug's licence in 1997 because a safer form became available.

Terfenadine (marketed as Triludan in the UK, and as Seldane in the US) came with a major black-box warning in bold capital letters in the US *Physicians' Desk Reference*. Interestingly, no such similar warning was published in the UK equivalent drugs 'bible', *The Data Sheet Compendium* (now *The Medicines Compendium*).

American doctors are warned that terfenadine can cause serious heart problems, including heart attack, irregular heart beat and *torsades de pointes*, when the heart beats abnormally fast. It is little wonder that this can sometimes end in a fatal attack.

These problems are magnified when terfenadine is taken with other drugs, including ketoconazole, itraconazole and erythromycin.

An early warning sign of an impending attack is often a fainting spell and a feeling of lightheadedness (a condition known as syncope).

The drug can also cause serious liver problems.

Overdosage can occur as low as 360 mg, which leaves little margin for error, as the recommended dose is one 60 mg tablet taken twice a day.

Along with the usual reactions of dizziness and drowsiness experienced with most antihistamines, terfenadine has also been reported to cause alopecia (hair loss or thinning), bronchospasms, confusion, depression, insomnia, mental disorders, nightmares, psoriasis, seizures and visual disturbances.

It's hardly surprising that, faced with that choice, most patients would prefer to take their chances with hayfever.

VIAGRA (sildenafil)
Treatment for impotence

Viagra is the stuff of urban myth. It also earned its manufacturer, Pfizer, a heap of money. Once approved by the US Food and Drug Administration, Viagra (sildenafil) quickly became one of the most successful drugs in the States, gaining an enormous amount of worldwide publicity along the way.

Viagra treats impotence, or penile dysfunction, as it is currently called. In just one week, a record 113,000 prescriptions were written out for it in America, compared with an average of 3,000 or so for any common or garden wonder drug. No wonder the drug has earned the nickname of 'Pfizer Riser' after the manufacturer.

So successful has the drug been that there is already a black market for it, and even some sexually active men are trying to get hold of the magic tablets just to improve their performance.

While some men are celebrating the belated return of their manhood, others would have a different story to tell—if they were alive to tell it. Six men died after taking the drug, and the Israeli health authority was the first to ban its introduction there, although it is not clear if the drug was directly responsible for the deaths.

A study of 532 men taking the drug revealed that reactions after short-term use included flushing, dyspepsia, visual disturbances and headache.

So, just when you're able to perform for the first time in ages, you're forced to call it off and you have to blame it on one of the oldest excuses in the book (N Engl J Med, 1998; 338: 1397–404).

VIOXX (rofecoxib)
Analgesic for arthritis

Vioxx (rofecoxib) is the first of a new kind of analgesic to be licensed in the UK. It employs a pioneering technology called COX-2 (selective cyclooygenase-2) inhibition, which is supposed to offer all the benefits of NSAIDs (non-steroidal anti-inflammatory drugs) such as aspirin and ibuprofen, but without damaging the stomach.

Although much of the breakthrough research is being carried out at Searle, the pharmaceutical company was beaten to the punch by Merck Sharp & Dohme (MSD), which succeeded in getting approval in the UK for Vioxx first.

In theory, the COX-2 inhibitor drugs can be used for any kind of pain relief, although MSD is marketing Vioxx as an antiarthritic.

But one party pooper, in the guise of the University of California, has already appeared on the scene. Researchers there doubt that the COX-2 drugs can protect your gastric lining after all and believe it may even induce ulcers (BMJ, 1999; 319: 1518).

Worse has since followed. It has now been linked to a non-bacterial form of meningitis. Seven cases have been reported in America, although none has been fatal.

In its own datasheet for the drug, MSD reveals that, in a trial of 5,400 people, more than one in 100 complained of heartburn, dyspepsia, nausea and diarrhoea, suggesting that the Californian researchers may be on to something. Other common adverse reactions included abdominal pain, dizziness, fluid retention, hypertension, headache and itching.

Less common reactions, reported by more than one in 1,000, included chest pains, acid reflux, constipation, oral ulcers, vomiting, tinnitus, weight gain, cramps, insomnia, vertigo, depression and dermatitis.

XENICAL (orlistat)
Weight-loss therapy

Xenical (orlistat) is a drug that is described by its manufacturer, Roche, as the 'fat controller'. Roche is not trying to muscle in on the magical world of children's stories, but is attempting a 'magic bullet' approach to weight control, presumably for those built like Thomas the Tank.

The approach is simple enough. If you're dangerously obese, just take Xenical, radically change your diet from a high fat one to one rich in fruit and vegetables, and—hey presto!—you'll lose weight. Proof positive that the drug works!

Of course, such a powerful drug with proven benefits doesn't come without some side effects. Most of them are gastrointestinal and socially embarrassing, such as flatus discharge, which is medical-speak for breaking wind with interest, "oily evacuations" and increased defecation.

But the problems don't end there. You could also develop tooth disorders, upper and lower respiratory infections, influenza, headache, menstrual irregularity, anxiety, fatigue and urinary tract infection.

One worry is that Xenical may not be tolerated if the patient is also taking an antidiabetic drug. As many obese people are also diabetics, this could be a major problem, and one that needs to be monitored carefully by your GP.

Roche is very exact about who should be prescribed Xenical. It should be given only to those who've tried to diet but failed to lose more than 2.5 kg (5.5 lb) over four weeks. Treatment should be stopped if the patient doesn't reduce his or her weight by more than 5 per cent over a 12-week treatment period.

If all this has put you off, you could just try instead the diet recommended by Roche to accompany the drug treatment. All those Thomas the Tanks might just become the Little Trains That Could . . .

ZANTAC (ranitidine)
Heartburn and ulcer drug

Zantac (ranitidine), the ulcer drug, was one of the world's top bestsellers until scientists discovered that most ulcers were caused by the *Helicobacter pylori* bug and could be successfully treated with antibiotics.

Glaxo has been advertising Zantac to treat ulcers caused by non-steroidal anti-inflammatory drugs (NSAIDs), painkillers mainly used for arthritis, before they've even appeared. A recent ad in the BMJ read: "Successfully healing both duodenal and gastric ulcers . . . used as prophylaxis [that is, just-in-case treatment], Zantac can actually prevent NSAID-associated duodenal ulcers. In fact, it's the only [ulcer drug] licensed to do this."

This raised the hackles of Findlay M. Hickley, the pharmaceutical prescribing advisor to the Grampian Health Board in Aberdeen, Scotland, who pointed out that the most likely site of damage caused by NSAIDs is the stomach mucosa, not the small intestine (duodenum).

He notes that the *British National Formulary* states: "Therapy [with H_2 antagonists] can promote the healing of NSAID-associated ulcers, but there is no proof that the ulcer complications [such as bleeding or perforation] are prevented."

He also notes that Zantac is only licensed as a just-in-case remedy against duodenal ulcers, not stomach ones (BMJ, 20/27 August 1994).

Needless to say, Glaxo replied that the ad doesn't actually say that it can prevent gastric ulcers (although the first part of the ad clearly suggests that it can by implication).

This use of an H_2 antagonist is of concern because some acid-blocking drugs are being released for sale over the counter.

Zantac is also being prescribed for heartburn.

If you're contemplating using this drug to control stomach side effects from NSAIDs, you should know that Zantac can cause nausea, vomiting, abdominal discomfort and pain.

ZESTRIL (lisinopril)
Hypertension and heart failure therapy
As its name implies, Zestril is supposed to put the spring back into the step of the elderly by treating high blood pressure and heart failure. Marketed by Zeneca, it is one of the powerful ACE inhibitors, and so comes with a range of side effects that may make any steps rather more faltering.

The common side effects include hypotension, or low blood pressure, and because of that, dizziness and headaches. Other likely reactions include diarrhoea, cough, nausea and fatigue.

Another concern can be angioedema, where vascular tissues fill with fluids, causing swelling. In most cases, the swelling goes down once the treatment is stopped, but emergency care needs to be given if the swelling is blocking the airways or affects the tongue or larynx.

Ironically, one reaction can be heart attack, the very thing the drug is supposed to prevent, although this is a rarer occurrence. Other less common reactions include abdominal pain, dry mouth, hepatitis, jaundice, mood swings, mental confusion, acute kidney failure and impotence.

People on the drug who suddenly develop a non-productive cough or a skin rash can be almost certain that it has been caused by the treatment, and the symptoms disappear once it is stopped.

Any cautious doctor should begin treatment with just 2.5 mg daily, which the manufacturer says is too little to have any beneficial effect, but should show any adverse reactions. The usual dose range is 10–20 mg a day, and the maximum recommended amount is 40 mg. The dose should be increased over a two- to four-week period. Any treatment must begin in hospital.

Because of its possible effects on the kidneys, patients who already suffer kidney problems should naturally enough not take the drug, or any other ACE inhibitor. As studies have never been carried out on children or nursing mothers, neither group is advised to start treatment.

ZIMOVANE (zopiclone)
Insomnia and anxiety therapy
Ever since benzodiazepines lost their favoured position as a safe treatment for insomnia and anxiety, the pharmaceutical industry has been frantically trying to fill the lucrative gap with a drug that does not cause dependence.

One likely candidate has been Zimovane (zopiclone), whose acceptance by doctors has been helped by claims from the manufacturer that "the risk of dependence is minimal when the duration of treatment is limited to no more than four weeks" (*The Data Sheet Compendium*, 1997, now called *The*

Medicines Compendium). Unfortunately, many patients take the drug for far longer than four weeks, in which case, the outcome can be very different, as two senior doctors at the University of Wales have reported.

In a report to the British Medical Journal, Drs Ian Jones and Gary Sullivan cited four cases at their hospital where patients suffered adverse reactions including severe anxiety, palpitations, sweating and tremors when they tried to come off the drug after taking it for a year or less (BMJ, 1998; 316: 117). One patient, a 49-year-old man, said he suffered a strong craving for the drug after he finished the treatment.

Other reactions can include depression, rebound insomnia, where the drug causes the very problem it is supposed to ease, and amnesia. Common reactions include having a metallic aftertaste in the mouth, stomach disturbances including nausea and vomiting, dizziness, headaches, drowsiness and dry mouth.

The University of Wales doctors believe that zopiclone should be used only as a short-term therapy. "It would seem reasonable to apply the same caution to prescribing this drug that is applied to the benzodiazepines."

Not exactly the message that the manufacturer wanted to hear. So . . . back to the drawing board?

ZOCOR (simvastatin)
Cholesterol-lowering therapy

Medicine is always on the lookout for a wonder drug that can miraculously tackle anything it's put up against. Take aspirin, for instance, a painkiller that became the cure-all of the century, with claims that it could prevent heart problems and a range of other conditions. Even thalidomide, the Richard Nixon of the drugs world, is coming back in from the cold as a miracle worker.

The latest candidates for universal invincibility are the statins, originally designed to lower cholesterol levels, and one of the most prescribed family of drugs in the world.

Several doctors have postulated that statins can help treat osteoporosis in women (Lancet, 2000; 355: 2185–8), while another group maintains that statins can reduce the risk of stroke in patients with heart disease (N Engl J Med, 2000; 343: 317–26). Heart patients may also benefit from statins because the drug can help promote the growth of new blood vessels, a team from the St Elizabeth's Medical Center in Boston has found (Nature Med, 2000; 6: 1004–10).

These findings are controversial, and they haven't met with approval from all quarters; one doctor has argued that, if the statins really could help the growth of blood vessels, they would also cause malignancies.

There's certainly no indication that they do that, but there's plenty else the statins can cause, judging by the side effects of one, Zocor 80 (simvastatin). Common reactions include abdominal pain, constipation, flatulence and headache. Less common are nausea, rash, alopecia, dizziness, muscle cramps, myalgia, vomiting and anaemia.

Consultants at Guy's Hospital in London noted that five men with coronary artery disease became impotent within a week of starting on the drug. Others became lethargic and suffered inertia.

Problems of impotence have never been picked up in various marketing trials, but are being noted by doctors whose patients begin the treatment.

Of course, Zocor's manufacturer points out, the important thing is to change your diet if you want to reduce cholesterol levels. Trouble is, being that responsible is at the other end of the spectrum from the miracle cure-all that medicine, and its patients, seem to crave.

ZORAC (tazarotene)
Psoriasis treatment

If you're a psoriasis sufferer, chances are you've been offered Zorac (tazarotene). It's one of the first retinoids (a vitamin A derivative) that can be applied directly to the skin. As such, it's being marketed heavily by its manufacturer, Allergan, as a successful treatment of mild-to-moderate plaque psoriasis.

One important element of its marketing are the results of a study involving 300 patients given 0.1 per cent or 0.05 per cent tazarotene gel once a day, or the steroid cream fluocinonide twice a day.

Overall improvement was similar among the treatments, but fewer of the tazarotene groups suffered a relapse 12 weeks after the therapy had finished. Although as a gel it's easy to apply, it also seems to be less well tolerated than some of its competitors. More of those in the tazarotene groups had to drop out because of side effects, which included irritation, burning and erythema (skin reddening) (J Am Acad Dermatol, 1998; 38: 705–11).

To this can be added the adverse reactions noted in earlier trials, such as pruritus (itching), experienced by up to a quarter of all patients, and a worsening of the psoriasis, which was reported by up to 10 per cent of all patients.

Not surprisingly, reaction is associated with higher concentrations of the gel. The higher-concentration gel of 0.1 per cent can cause up to 5 per cent more cases of severe skin irritation than the lower concentration gel, especially during the first four weeks of use, the manufacturer warns.

Pregnant women and breastfeeding mothers should not use the gel, nor should any woman who is thinking of becoming pregnant. Its safety in patients under the age of 18 has not been proven.

ZOTON (lansoprazole)
Reflux and heartburn remedy

It's pretty unusual for any drug to be hailed as "the people's champion", but that's the claim being made for lansoprazole, an antiulcer treatment marketed in the UK as Zoton and in the US as Prevacid.

To back this claim, the marketers explain that "more doctors are turning to Zoton . . . Zoton is now on 85 per cent of UK hospital formularies."

So, for "people's champion", read "doctors' champion." And the reason why doctors are turning to it is because, after just two weeks of treatment, Zoton "relieves significantly more symptoms than omeprazole".

Zoton is designed to treat gastroesophageal reflux disease (GORD) and duodenal ulcer. It is also designed to treat symptoms associated with reflux, such as heartburn.

As such, it's a little surprising that it's so successful among doctors, particularly following the discovery of the ulcer-causing *Helicobacter pylori* bug. To be fair, it has been tested as a dual therapy with an antibiotic, and was effective in treating the bug and preventing its recurrence.

Similarly, it's been a successful treatment for heartburn, but terms involving words such as "sledgehammer" and "nut" come to mind, particularly when you look at the litany of possible side effects.

Ironically, these include gastrointestinal disturbances (that's right, the very thing it is supposedly treating), taste disturbances, malaise, headache and dizziness.

More serious, but rarer, reactions have included myalgia (muscle pain), depression, hallucinations, vertigo, jaundice, hepatitis, impotence, hair thinning and blurred vision.

Serious skin reactions are also rare, but have included rashes, says the manufacturer.

As usual, nursing mothers and children should not be taking the drug.

ZOVIRAX (aciclovir)

Herpes and shingles treatment

Amid all the bad publicity for AZT, aciclovir (or Zovirax, as it is known by its brand name) is Wellcome's big success story.

This antiviral drug inhibits a variety of human herpesviruses, including herpes simplex type 1 (cold sores) and type 2 (the genital variety) as well as varicella–zoster virus (the cause of shingles), Epstein–Barr virus and cytomegalovirus.

The non-prescription topical version (a less potent form of the drug) is known as the drug that beat cold sores, propelling it forward as the company's bestseller. Indeed, aciclovir is most effective against herpes type 1, and has a decreasing efficacy against the other viral infections in the order in which they appear above.

The drug works by inhibiting viral DNA replication and terminating DNA. When used for genital herpes, double-blind, placebo-controlled studies have showed that orally administered aciclovir significantly reduced the durations of acute infection, pain and new lesion formation, and also the frequency and severity of recurrences, in more than 95 per cent of patients.

In another study, almost half the patients remained free of recurrences in the first year and nearly two-thirds by the third year.

This, of course, entails taking the drug continuously over that time.

As for shingles, scientific studies of 187 patients showed that the drug shortened the durations of lesions, scabbing, healing and pain. A recent study showed no benefit of long-term Zovirax therapy with or without steroids over seven-day treatment with Zovirax alone (N Engl J Med, 31 March 1994).

The biggest problem is with chronic use of aciclovir. This can lead to the development of resistant viruses that will no longer respond to the drug. Furthermore, animal studies have shown that Zovirax can cause decreased production of sperm in males and, in females, cause implantation difficulties, leading to infertility, and also possible chromosomal mutations and birth defects.

Wellcome cautions that the drug shouldn't be taken by pregnant women or nursing mothers.

The most frequent adverse reactions were headache, numbness and tingling, general muscle weakness and pain, vomiting, diarrhoea, dizziness, anorexia, swelling, leg pain, swollen glands in the groin and lowered white blood cell counts.

LIST OF DRUGS

ZYDOL (tramadol hydrochloride)

Analgesic

If a drug is found to cause a serious adverse reaction not noted in early trials, doctors are sent a 'Dear Doctor' letter from the drug regulators to warn them of the new discovered dangers.

But, of course, it's a system that only works if the doctor actually reads the letter. Take, for instance, the case of the analgesic drug tramadol hydrochloride (marketed in the UK as Zydol, and as Ultram in the US).

Within a year of its approval in the US in 1995, 83 reports of seizures among tramadol patients were reported to the American drug regulator, the Food and Drug Administration (FDA).

So a 'Dear Doctor' letter was issued to all practitioners in the US and, in the following year, the number of reported cases rocketed to 200!

The American drug 'bible', *Physicians' Drug Reference*, also has warnings of seizures plastered across it which, again, seem to have gone unread. UK doctors have the perfect excuse, by the way, because their drug bible, *The Data Sheet Compendium* (now *The Medicines Compendium*), hardly mentions anything about seizures at all.

Seizures tend to occur within one day of taking the drug, and usually after taking 400 mg or less of tramadol a day. Seizure victims tend to be young and healthy people, aged between 20 and 39 years, and without any previous history of seizure.

But if you're lucky enough to escape seizures, the drug does come with other surprises. Serious, and sometimes fatal, anaphylactic (allergic) shock has been reported in patients, but the most common side effects include dizziness and vertigo, nausea, constipation, headache and vomiting.

We just thought we'd better tell you as your doctor probably won't have read about it.